Essentials of laparoscopy

DATE DUE

SEP 0 2 1997		
NOV 2 9 1997		
FEB 1 6 1998		
AUG 2 8 1998		
FEB 0 2 1999		
FEB 0 8 1999		
AUG 1 7 1999		
MAR 0 2 2000		
AUG 1 7 2000		
SEP 0 8 2000		
NOV 1 4 03		

DEMCO 38-297

ESSENTIALS OF
Laparoscopy

EDITED BY

Nathaniel J. Soper, M.D.
Associate Professor of Surgery
Division of Gastrointestinal Surgery
Washington University School of Medicine
St. Louis, Missouri

Randall R. Odem, M.D.
Assistant Professor of Obstetrics and Gynecology
Division of Reproductive Endocrinology
Washington University School of Medicine
St. Louis, Missouri

Ralph V. Clayman, M.D.
Professor of Urology and Radiology
Washington University School of Medicine
St. Louis, Missouri

Elspeth M. McDougall, M.D.
Assistant Professor of Urology
Washington University School of Medicine
St. Louis, Missouri

with 256 illustrations

QUALITY MEDICAL PUBLISHING, INC

ST. LOUIS, MISSOURI   1994

Every effort has been made to ensure the accuracy of the drug dosages listed in this book; however, the health care professional is legally responsible for verifying the indications and dosage requirements with the manufacturers' package inserts and is thus advised.

PUBLISHER   Karen Berger

PROJECT MANAGER   Suzanne Seeley Wakefield

PRODUCTION   Judy Bamert

DESIGN   Diane Beasley Design

COVER ART   Floyd E. Hosmer, Certified Medical Illustrator

Quality Medical Publishing, Inc.
11970 Borman Drive, Suite 222
St. Louis, Missouri 63146

LIBRARY OF CONGRESS CATALOGING-IN-PUBLICATION DATA

Essentials of laparoscopy / Nathaniel J. Soper . . . [et al.].
    p.   cm.
    Includes bibliographical references and index.
    ISBN 0-942219-53-8
    1. Abdomen—Endoscopic surgery.   I. Soper, Nathaniel J.
    [DNLM: 1. Laparoscopy—methods.   2. Surgery, Laparoscopic.   WI
575 E78 1994]
    RD540.E73   1994
    617.5′5059—dc20
    DNLM/DLC
    for Library of Congress   93-27517
                                                                        CIP

GW/M/M
5   4   3   2   1

To

or families and *our patients*

in hopes of creating a kinder,
gentler tomorrow

■

In the time of your life, live—
so that in that wondrous time you shall
not add to the misery and sorrow of the world,
but shall smile to the infinite delight
and mystery of it.

William Saroyan

Contributors

David M. Albala, M.D.
Assistant Professor of Urology, Loyola University Medical Center,
Chicago, Ilinois

Paramjit S. Chandoke, M.D.
Assistant Professor of Surgery, Division of Urology, Colorado Health
Sciences Center, Denver, Colorado

David S. Goldstein, M.D.
Resident in Urology, Harvard Medical School,
Boston, Massachusetts

Louis R. Kavoussi, M.D.
Assistant Professor of Urology, Johns Hopkins University,
Baltimore, Maryland

Diane F. Merritt, M.D.
Associate Professor of Obstetrics and Gynecology, Division of
Reproductive Endocrinology, Washington University School of Medicine, St.
Louis, Missouri

Terri G. Monk, M.D.
Assistant Professor of Anesthesiology, Washington University School
of Medicine, St Louis, Missouri

William A. See, M.D.
Assistant Professor of Urology, University of Iowa School of Medicine,
Iowa City, Iowa

B. Craig Weldon, M.D.
Instructor in Anesthesiology, Washington University School of Medicine,
St. Louis, Missouri

Howard N. Winfield, M.D.
Associate Professor of Urology, University of Iowa School of Medicine,
Iowa City, Iowa

Preface

Laparoscopy, or the examination of the abdominal cavity by means of an endoscope, is not new, having been first performed in 1901. Initially this technique was used only for visual examination of the peritoneal cavity. Subsequently auxiliary trocars were introduced; through these, instruments could be inserted to perform laparoscopically guided biopsies. During the 1970s the pioneering efforts of engineer-gynecologist Kurt Semm in Germany showed that "pelviscopic surgery" was a possibility. He designed many instruments and devised techniques that facilitated laparoscopic surgery and rendered many basic maneuvers safe. Advances in optics and fiberoptic light transmission improved the laparoscopic images, but it was not until video technology was harnessed to the laparoscope that the surgeon's eye was freed from the monocular laparoscopic eyepiece, and all members of the operating team were able to observe procedures simultaneously from the same viewpoint. The first laparoscopic cholecystectomies were performed by E. Muhe of Böblingen, Germany (1985) and P. Mouret of Lyon, France (1987). Dissemination of the procedure gained momentum when it crossed the Atlantic Ocean, setting in motion a "revolution" in surgery whereby tens of thousands of general surgeons have been trained in basic laparoscopic techniques; likewise, urologists and gynecologists have been reawakened to the expanding possibilities of laparoscopic surgery.

The startling clarity of video laparoscopic images, combined with an increasing familiarity with laparoscopic manipulation of tissue experienced by thousands of surgeons, ensured that some individuals would begin improvising and trying to expand the applications of laparoscopic operations. With the rapid acceptance of laparoscopic surgery and the pace at which surgeons were trained in laparoscopic techniques, it is not surprising that a number of complications arising from laparoscopic surgery have occurred. It is important, therefore, to ensure that the basics of laparoscopy are performed in a standardized, safe fashion.

Essentials of Laparoscopy is intended to prepare the neophyte surgeon for performing laparoscopy in a practical, straightforward, step-by-step manner. This book concentrates on the basic techniques, instrumentation, and complications unique to laparoscopy. As such, it is specifically designed for those surgeons who are either unfamiliar with or just beginning laparoscopy, both at the resident and postgraduate level. In addition, many surgeons already trained in laparoscopic surgery may benefit by reviewing the detailed chapters covering each aspect of basic laparoscopy. Within this book are more than 250 original line drawings specifically designed to clarify each laparoscopic principle. The book is purposely sized to fit within the pocket of a laboratory coat and has a special "lay-flat" binding and large, easy-to-read print. In every respect, we have endeavored to make the text user friendly. Quite simply, this textbook is meant to be read and reread.

If the principles outlined within these pages are learned and applied, the fear and failure of laparoscopy will be adverted—much to the delight of the surgeon and patient alike. To this end, the contents of this volume go straight to the core of the surgical craft: *Primum non nocere.*

Acknowledgments

We would all like to acknowledge the untiring, yeomanly efforts of Suzanne Wakefield and Judy Bamert, without whom this project would have remained just another "good idea" that never came to fruition.

Nathaniel J. Soper
Randall R. Odem
Ralph V. Clayman
Elspeth M. McDougall

Contents

ESSENTIALS OF
Laparoscopy

CHAPTER 1

Selection and Preparation of the Patient for Laparoscopic Surgery

William A. See and Nathaniel J. Soper

PATIENT SELECTION: RELATIVE CONTRAINDICATIONS TO LAPAROSCOPY

An adequate history and physical examination remain the cornerstone of patient selection (see boxes, pp. 2 and 3). Relative and absolute contraindications to laparoscopic surgery may be identified from the history, physical examination, and initial laboratory studies. In addition to these problems specific to the laparoscopic procedure, preexisting conditions that place the patient at risk for anesthesia-related complications (i.e., severe cardiac or pulmonary disease) must be considered.

Prior abdominal/pelvic surgery Prior abdominal surgery constitutes the most commonly encountered relative contraindication to laparoscopy. The nature of the procedure, the location of the previous incision, and the location of the planned laparoscopic procedure must be integrated into the overall risk/benefit analysis. Depending on the location of the prior procedure, it may be possible to insert the Veress needle

1

Prelaparoscopy patient history checklist

Past medical history

☐ Enumeration of each prior abdominal/pelvic surgical procedure and the underlying etiology (e.g., peritonitis secondary to a ruptured appendix)

☐ Abdominal radiation: reason and exact placement of the radiation therapy portals

☐ Intra-abdominal or pelvic inflammation or infection (e.g., generalized peritonitis, cholecystitis, diverticulitis, endometriosis, peptic ulcer disease, pelvic inflammatory disease)

☐ Hip prosthesis (retroperitoneal leakage of prosthetic glue may result in extreme pelvic fibrosis)

☐ Other prosthetic or cardiac problems indicating a need for subacute bacterial endocarditis prevention

☐ Prior deep venous thrombosis or history of thromboembolic disorders

Risk factors for general anesthesia

☐ Significant pulmonary or cardiac disease

☐ Prior anesthetic problems

☐ Hypertension (? controlled)

Medications

☐ Steroids

☐ Pulmonary medications

☐ Cardiac medications

☐ Anticoagulants or agents with an anticoagulant effect (e.g., aspirin, nonsteroidal anti-inflammatory agents)

Allergies

☐ Medications (including local anesthetics)

☐ Skin preparations (e.g., Betadine)

and primary working port trocar at sites away from abdominal wall adhesions (Chapter 4). Alternatively, the minilaparotomy approach, with the open (e.g., Hasson) cannula, may be used to allow primary trocar insertion under direct vision (Chapter 5). We have found that once a primary telescopic port and secondary working port have been inserted, relatively extensive adhesiolysis may be safely undertaken to facilitate subsequent port positioning.

Prelaparoscopy physical examination checklist

General
- ☐ Blood pressure: rule out uncontrolled hypertension
- ☐ Temperature: rule out sepsis
- ☐ Pulse: rule out uncorrected cardiac dysrhythmias

Chest and cardiac examination
- ☐ Routine examination to determine suitability for a general anesthetic

Abdominal and pelvic examination
Inspection
- ☐ Site of prior incisions
- ☐ Umbilical abnormalities
- ☐ Umbilical hernia
- ☐ Incisional hernia

Palpation
- ☐ Intra-abdominal mass
- ☐ Abdominal tenderness: localized, general/deep, or rebound
- ☐ Umbilical hernia
- ☐ Incisional hernia
- ☐ Widened aortic pulsation (rule out abdominal aortic aneurysm)
- ☐ Fixed or frozen pelvis on vaginal/rectal examination

Auscultation
- ☐ Bruits indicative of aortic or iliac/femoral artery aneurysms
- ☐ Bowel sounds (rule out obstruction)

Previous peritonitis or pelvic fibrosis   Patients with a history of pelvic or intra-abdominal infection (i.e., peritonitis) may be suboptimal candidates for laparoscopy. In this regard a careful history is essential to discern the indication for each abdominal or pelvic surgical procedure that the patient has previously undergone. A ruptured appendix or disrupted colonic diverticulum results in significant scarring and a large number of adhesions. If these patients are to undergo a laparoscopic procedure, the Veress needle must be placed as far as possible from the site of the affected organ or surgical site (Chapter 4). The surgeon must anticipate that a significant part of the procedure will be involved with the lysis of the adhesions.

Obesity Obesity is another commonly encountered relative contraindication to laparoscopy. The associated increase in thickness of the anterior abdominal wall makes the establishment of the pneumoperitoneum and trocar introduction more difficult. In certain patients the sheer mass of the anterior abdominal wall may necessitate the maintenance of higher insufflation pressures (20 mm Hg) to obtain an adequate working space in the peritoneal cavity. Additional difficulties in obese patients include a diminished ability to transilluminate the abdominal wall in order to avoid injury to the superficial abdominal wall vessels when placing additional trocars. Once the pneumoperitoneum is established and trocar introduction achieved, the procedure may be further hampered by large amounts of both intraperitoneal and pelvic adipose tissues. Also, the thicker abdominal wall ($\geq$14 cm versus 6 cm in a normal individual) further impedes the maneuverability of the laparoscopic ports necessary to gain access to various areas of the abdomen. Finally, the fasciotomy of the larger port sites (i.e., $\geq$10 mm) usually cannot be closed in an obese patient. Hence such a patient will be predisposed to a potentially increased risk of herniation at a trocar site unless staples or sutures are used to at least close the peritoneal cavity from the inside.

Unreducible abdominal/inguinal hernia In patients with *unreducible* herniations of the abdominal contents, the pneumoperitoneum may result in vascular compromise of the incarcerated viscus.

Umbilical abnormalities Before any laparoscopic procedure, the umbilicus should be examined carefully. Evidence of an umbilical hernia, presence of a urachal remnant, or a history of an umbilical herniorrhaphy precludes the use of the umbilicus as the primary site for placement of the Veress needle.

The history may contain evidence of the rare patient with symptoms of vestigial infraumbilical midline structures. Any history of umbilical discharge should prompt the surgeon to order diagnostic studies to exclude urachal cysts or sinuses before the performance of laparoscopy. This problem, if recognized preoperatively, can be overcome by choosing a lateral site on the abdomen for insufflation.

Abdominal aortic/iliac aneurysm During the physical examination, careful palpation and auscultation of the abdomen are important to determine the presence of an abdominal or aortic/iliac artery aneurysm.

If the findings suggest this diagnosis, an ultrasound examination should be obtained to evaluate both the aorta and iliac vessels. These patients are obviously at increased risk for vascular injury during Veress needle placement and trocar introduction. Vascular consultation for repair of this problem should be seriously considered before laparoscopic surgery. If one elects to proceed with laparoscopy in these patients, an upper quadrant site for passage of the Veress needle should be selected.

Severe pulmonary disease   The patient with marked pulmonary compromise is at a significantly increased risk for complications arising from laparoscopic surgery. The pressure of the pneumoperitoneum restricts ventilation. Furthermore, the head-down position commonly necessary for many pelvic procedures further increases the pressure on the diaphragm, thereby decreasing its excursion. Also, the accumulation of CO_2 during the procedure and the development of hypercarbia necessitate hyperventilation to preclude the development of an associated acidosis. As discussed in Chapter 3, the exhaled concentration of CO_2 may cause underestimation of arterial levels of CO_2, thereby lulling the surgeon and anesthesiologist into a false sense of security. In these patients, helium or another inert gas may be substituted for CO_2 thereby precluding hypercarbia and its associated acidosis.

Bowel obstruction   Obstruction of the bowel with distended loops of small and/or large intestine increases the risk of injury to the hollow viscera during initial entry of the laparoscopic trocars into the abdominal cavity. Moreover, the presence of the distended intestine may preclude adequate visualization and diminish the effective working space within the pneumoperitoneum. Before operating on patients with suspected bowel obstruction or ileus, a nasogastric tube should be placed and the bowel decompressed as much as possible. Entry into the abdominal cavity may be most safely afforded by a direct cutdown ("open cannula") technique as described in Chapter 5.

Pregnancy   Pregnancy is a relative contraindication, and its presence requires added precautions in the care of the mother and fetus. Indications include general diagnostic laparoscopy as well as therapeutic disorders of the ovary, appendix, and gallbladder. The general diagnosis and management of these problems in pregnancy is at times different from that of a patient in the nonpregnant state, and these issues are discussed elsewhere. Elective procedures are contraindicated during pregnancy; however, when the decision is made that surgery is needed, the early second trimester is the preferable period. Because placement of an intrauterine manipulator is contraindicated, the procedure is best performed with the patient in a supine position (Fig. 1-1). One should consider use of pneumatic intermittent compression boots, a Foley catheter, and stomach drainage via an orogastric tube. Standard inhalation anesthesia with controlled ventilation and monitoring of end-tidal CO_2 is appropriate. Doppler examination of fetal heart tones is mandatory preoperatively, after induction of anesthesia, and in the immediate postoperative period. Intraoperative fetal monitoring is not feasible because of the space that develops between the abdominal wall and the uterus from the pneumoperitoneum.

A pregnant patient may require alternative approaches in establishing a pneumoperitoneum. This may include use of open laparoscopy (see Chapter 5) or an alternative insertion site to prevent injury to the uterus (Fig. 1-2). The fundus of the uterus lies immediately below the

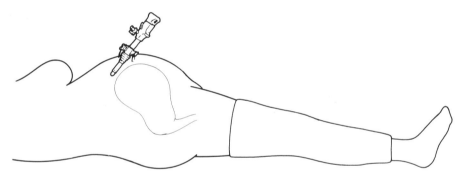

Fig. 1-1 The supine position is preferable for laparoscopy in a pregnant patient. Uterine manipulators are not used. Use of pneumatic intermittent compression boots, as shown, should be considered.

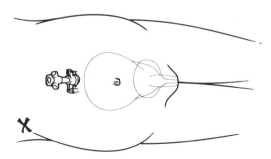

Fig. 1-2 Great care should be taken to avoid injury to the pregnant uterus. This would usually mandate open laparoscopy. Care must be taken to avoid contact with this sheath and the uterus. One may also consider an alternative site for trocar insertion (X).

umbilicus at 20 weeks' gestation, and care must be taken to avoid injury to the pregnant uterus. When using open laparoscopy one must also remember the potential for damage from the operative sheath to this enlarged abdominal organ. Care must also be taken to maximize blood flow to the pregnant uterus. As pregnancy progresses beyond the middle of the second trimester, one must become more concerned with maintaining a left lateral decubitus location of the uterus.

There are minimal data available concerning the effect of prolonged CO_2 pneumoperitoneum on fetal physiology. Intuitively, prolonged absorption of carbon dioxide could lead to fetal respiratory acidosis. Placental removal of fetal CO_2 occurs rapidly and represents minimal potential problems. Nevertheless, close monitoring of end-tidal CO_2 is warranted, and the intra-abdominal pressure should be maintained at less than 12 mm Hg.

In summary, pregnancy is a relative contraindication to laparoscopy and may be considered by an experienced surgeon who is capable of performing procedures expeditiously. The performance of these procedures should be done only after consultation with and full agreement from the woman's primary obstetrician.

In this regard, Soper and colleagues have performed laparoscopic cholecystectomies on six severely symptomatic pregnant women and have had no complications to date. Each patient delivered a healthy infant at term. They limited intervention to the *second* trimester of gestation. To prevent inadvertent injury to the uterus, an open insertion of the initial port or alternative site of insertion in one of the upper abdominal quadrants should be used. The mothers were hyperventilated, and close monitoring of the end-tidal CO_2 and *arterial* CO_2 was undertaken to prevent fetal acidosis. For each patient, perioperative consultation with an obstetrician specializing in high-risk cases was sought. Perioperative monitoring of fetal heart tones is important, including transvaginal monitoring during the procedure itself. In pregnant patients, the insufflation pressure is kept at <12 mm Hg to prevent respiratory problems or decreased vena caval return.

PATIENT SELECTION: ABSOLUTE CONTRAINDICATIONS TO LAPAROSCOPY

There are four absolute contraindications to laparoscopy: *generalized peritonitis*, an *uncorrected coagulopathy*, *inability to tolerate a laparotomy*, and an *inexperienced surgeon*. First, establishing a pneumoperitoneum in the face of generalized peritonitis presents the risk of dissemination of the infectious processes and will probably only delay the inevitable open laparotomy necessary to resolve the underlying problem. Next, any laparoscopic intervention is fraught with hazard when an uncorrectable or uncorrected coagulopathy is encountered, because brisk hemorrhage is more difficult to control using laparoscopic techniques than with an open operative field.

Laparoscopic control of hemorrhage is limited when accumulated blood obscures sites of hemorrhage or splashes on the laparoscopic lens and when smoke or vapor generated by thermal instrument sources diminish visualization. The ability to aspirate blood from the peritoneal cavity is limited by the finite luminal diameter of the aspiration probes introduced through 5 mm or 10 mm laparoscopic sheaths and by the sudden decrease in the visual field as a result of the application of aspiration to the pneumoperitoneum-induced working space. Also, it is more difficult to stem hemorrhage by direct pressure using laparoscopic techniques. Therefore coagulopathies must be reversed before a laparoscopic procedure is undertaken.

Finally, the patient must be in a state of health sufficient to tolerate a laparotomy—and the surgeon must be in a sufficient state of training to successfully perform the procedure. Just because one is operating through a "small hole" does not mean that laparoscopy is not "big time" surgery, replete with all and more of the potentially fatal complications associated with open surgical procedures.

PATIENT PREPARATION

Obtaining informed consent by thoroughly discussing the risks, benefits, alternatives to, and potential complications of laparoscopy is the initial step in preparing the patient for laparoscopic intervention. This should result in a clear understanding by the patient of the potential need for open surgical intervention (see Appendix C). The patient *must consent* to an open surgical procedure should the laparoscopy result in an emergency situation (e.g., hemorrhage or bowel or bladder injury).

Depending on the nature of the procedure and an assessment of the patient's individual risk for bowel injury (e.g., prior abdominal surgery), mechanical or full bowel preparation may be given the day before the procedure. For simple diagnostic or routine outpatient procedures (e.g., tubal ligation) a bowel preparation is not necessary. However, if the beginning laparoscopist wishes to decompress the bowels before a simple diagnostic or planned pelvic procedure, bowel preparation can be simplified to a full liquid diet (excluding dairy products) for 48 hours before the procedure and the administration of 10 oz of magnesium citrate 48 hours before the planned procedure. For longer therapeutic procedures some institutions routinely order an outpatient bowel preparation for maximal decompression of the bowels. Also, by giving a

Bowel preparation

- ☐ Two days before procedure: clear liquid diet
- ☐ The day before surgery: 4 L of chilled GoLYTELY or NuLYTELY PO until rectal effluent is clear (1 PM-6 PM)
- ☐ At 1 PM, 7 PM, and 11 PM: neomycin, 1 g PO/erythromycin base, 1 g PO
- ☐ NPO after 12 AM; IVs only
- ☐ Compazine, 10 mg PO, at 2 PM to stop nausea

complete outpatient bowel preparation, a primary repair can be accomplished if a bowel injury occurs. The box shows typical orders for bowel preparation.

Patients are advised to discontinue anticoagulants and any platelet-inhibiting medications (e.g., aspirin, nonsteroidal anti-inflammatory agents) at least 7 days before laparoscopy. If there is any question concerning the patient's coagulation status, a bleeding time should be obtained.

Routine laboratory studies are ordered before laparoscopy (e.g., evaluations of serum sodium, potassium, chloride, and bicarbonate and blood cell count). If there is a history of a bleeding diathesis, a coagulation battery is done (prothrombin time, partial thromboplastin time, and bleeding time). For older patients, a chest radiograph and electrocardiogram are obtained. Pulmonary evaluation (including pulmonary function tests and arterial blood gas determination) and cardiac stress tests may be appropriate in high-risk individuals.

If the procedure is of a diagnostic or a minor therapeutic nature, a type and screen are sufficient. Blood is typed and cross-matched before any major laparoscopic operation. In these cases the patient must be given the option of donating autologous blood or obtaining donor-directed units from family or friends.

Finally, broad-spectrum antibiotics should be administered intravenously before an incision is made in all patients who have the potential for bacterial contamination of the wound or abdominal cavity. In patients with no history of a penicillin allergy, the antibiotic of choice is generally a long-acting second-generation cephalosporin. In the absence of significant intraoperative contamination, the preoperative dose is considered to be adequate prophylaxis against postoperative septic complications.

CONCLUSION

Safe laparoscopic surgery hinges on successful completion of each step in the process, beginning with patient identification and concluding with appropriate follow-up. Careful patient selection and preparation are the critical initial steps in this sequence of events.

If it starts out wrong, it is not going to finish up right.

REFERENCES

1. Saleh JW. Laparoscopy. Philadelphia: WB Saunders, 1988.
2. Berci G, Cuschieri A. Practical Laparoscopy. London: Baillière Tindall, 1986.
3. Hulka JF. Textbook of Laparoscopy. Orlando, Fla.: Grune & Stratton, 1985.
4. Wolff BG, Beart RW Jr., Dozois RR, et al. A new bowel preparation for elective colon and rectal surgery: A prospective, randomized clinical trial. Arch Surg 123:895, 1988.
5. Soper NJ. Effect of nonbiliary problems impacting on laparoscopic cholecystectomy. Am J Surg 165:522-526, 1993.
6. Soper NJ, Hunter J, Petrie RH. Laparoscopic cholecystectomy in pregnancy. Surg Endosc 6:115-117, 1992.
7. Jackson SJ, Sigman HH. Laparoscopic cholecystectomy in pregnancy. J Laparoendoscop Surg 3:35, 1993.
8. Cherry SH, Berkowitz RL, Kase NG. Medical, Surgical, and Gynecologic Complications of Pregnancy, 3rd ed. Baltimore: Williams & Wilkins, 1985.

CHAPTER 2

Room Set-up and Patient Positioning

Ralph V. Clayman and Howard N. Winfield

ROOM SET-UP: GENERAL

Laparoscopic surgery is "technology intensive." Before any laparoscopic procedure is initiated, a checklist should be completed on the equipment essential for the procedure. All of the necessary equipment must be present and functioning before the patient arrives in the operating room. The middle of the procedure is no time to learn that the CO_2 tank is empty or that the irrigation solution has not been properly prepared or pressurized.

The box on pp. 12-13 provides a checklist that can be photocopied and placed in the laparoscopy suite. The surgeon should personally run through the checklist at the start of each laparoscopic case. Thus, *before* the patient has been anesthetized the surgeon should know that all essential equipment is present and operational. The box on pp. 13-16 provides a detailed list of equipment used during a basic laparoscopic procedure.

Laparoscopy: Operating room checklist for sterile equipment

Insufflation

- ☐ CO_2 tank full and spare tank available
- ☐ CO_2 line attached
- ☐ CO_2 coming through insufflator line (bubbles under water with a machine pressure <2 mm Hg)
- ☐ Pressure gauge working; when the insufflator line is kinked the registered pressure should rapidly rise to >15 mm Hg
- ☐ Flow shut-off working: with peak pressure set at 15 mm Hg, kinking the tubing should cause the flow of CO_2 to drop to 0 L/min

Camera/endoscope/video monitor/light source

- ☐ Light source operational and attached to laparoscope
- ☐ Sterile camera wrap in place over camera or camera sterilized
- ☐ Camera attached to 10 mm laparoscope
- ☐ Camera white-balanced (after attached to laparoscope)
- ☐ Camera focused
- ☐ Sharp, true color image on monitor

Irrigation/aspiration

- ☐ 1 L of lactated Ringer's solution or normal saline ($\pm$ 5000 units of heparin and 500 mg of cefazolin premixed)
- ☐ Biomedical dynamics pressure bag to pressurize solution to 250 mm Hg or a pressurized irrigation setup (e.g., Nezhat irrigator/aspirator)
- ☐ Irrigation flows rapidly through irrigator/aspirator (trumpet valve not plugged)
- ☐ Wall suction connected to suction line of irrigator/aspirator
- ☐ Fluid can readily be aspirated from a basin

Electrosurgical unit

- ☐ Grounding pad attached to patient
- ☐ Cord on the table and plugged into dissector
- ☐ Settings for coagulation and cutting current selected
- ☐ Insulation intact along entire shaft of electrosurgical instruments
- ☐ Foot pedal is placed next to surgeon's dominant foot

Laser units

- ☐ Turned on and pretested
- ☐ Appropriate setting selected
- ☐ Appropriate eye protection available for use
- ☐ Smoke evacuation system present and functional
- ☐ Laser warning sign for door

Laparoscopy: Operating room checklist for sterile equipment—cont'd

CO_2 laser

☐ Proper couplings available
☐ Operative laparoscopes or laser guides available
☐ Arm tucked to side
☐ Fine-focused HeNe beam

Fiberoptic lasers

☐ Laser fibers in room
☐ Fiber cleavers and strippers of same size as fiber to be utilized present in room
☐ Irrigation/aspiration channels in room
☐ Fiber diverter available

Patient

☐ Nasogastric or orogastric tube
☐ Foley catheter
☐ Scrotum wrapped (optional)
☐ Phallus wrapped (optional)
☐ Patient strapped to table; arms tucked at sides
☐ Compression stockings (+ / − pneumatic)

Other

☐ LAPAROTOMY SET

Room set-up checklist for laparoscopic surgery

Laparoscopic tray
Veress needle

☐ Disposable or reusable
☐ Check patency and function of spring on inner hollow stylet

Trocar-sheath units

☐ 5, 10, and 12 mm
☐ Disposable or reusable
☐ Open cannula (e.g., Hasson)

Laparoscope

☐ 10 mm: 0-degree lens
☐ 10 mm: 30-degree lens
☐ 5 mm: 0-degree lens

Continued.

Room set-up checklist for laparoscopic surgery—cont'd

Forceps

☐ Straight and curved (Maryland)—5 and 10 mm
☐ Atraumatic (insulated)
☐ Spoon-shaped tissue retrieval (10 mm)
☐ Toothed traumatic (insulated): locking and nonlocking types

Scissors

☐ Insulated straight
☐ Insulated curved (disposable)
☐ Serrated
☐ Hook

Electrosurgical instruments

☐ Corson needles
☐ Cutting spatula blade
☐ Curved scissors

Uterine manipulation instruments

☐ Open-sided speculum
☐ Tenaculum
☐ Uterine manipulator
☐ Dressing forceps

Hemostatic

☐ Multifire clip applicator
☐ Preformed ligature
☐ Laparoscopic needle driver
☐ Argon beam coagulator (optional)
☐ Avitene

Suction-irrigation unit

☐ Triple-lumen Luer Lock

Cords and tubings

☐ Cautery × 2
☐ Fiberoptic light cable
☐ Video camera chip unit
☐ Irrigation
☐ Suction
☐ CO_2

Room set-up checklist for laparoscopic surgery—cont'd

Retractors

☐ Fan
☐ Blunt tip

Miscellaneous

☐ Uterine manipulator/insufflator (for gynecologic procedures)
☐ Methylene blue insufflating fluid (for gynecologic procedures)
☐ Syringe, 10 cc, disposable
☐ Foley catheter, 16 Fr, 5 cc balloon
☐ Salem sump nasogastric tube, 16 Fr
☐ IV pressure infusion bag
☐ Laparoscopic lens antifog agent
☐ Scalpel with No. 10 and No. 15 blades
☐ Two towel clamps (large)
☐ Four hemostats
☐ Suture scissors
☐ Mayo Hegar needle holder
☐ Tissue forceps, heavy, 6 inches
☐ Semken tissue forceps
☐ Suture: PDS 2/0 SH
☐ Two Kocher clamps
☐ Two Sinn retractors

Laparoscopic basic equipment
CO_2 insufflator

☐ Adjustable high flow (1-10 L/min)
☐ Intraperitoneal pressure gauge
☐ Total CO_2 insufflated gauge

CO_2 source

☐ Wall unit
☐ Tank, regulator

Light source

☐ High intensity—xenon

Video system

☐ Two color TV monitors, high resolution
☐ Full-beam camera chip
☐ Video monitor
☐ ½-inch or ¾-inch tapes
☐ Video recorder
☐ Print monitor

Continued.

Room set-up checklist for laparoscopic surgery—cont'd

General equipment
☐ Operating table with multidirectional movements
☐ Electrosurgical machine with foot pedals and grounding pads
☐ Suction system
☐ Adhesive tape, 3-inch
☐ Foam pads and boots
☐ Counted sponges (10)
☐ Urimeter
☐ Preparation tray
☐ Stirrups, stirrup clamps, stirrup pads

Laparotomy set-up
☐ MUST BE IN OR THEATER FOR EMERGENCY USE

PATIENT PREPARATION

Once the patient is in the operating room, an orogastric or nasogastric tube and pneumatic compression stockings are placed (Fig. 2-1), and a urethral catheter is inserted. The goal is to drain any intra-abdominal or pelvic viscus before insertion of the Veress needle. In this regard the full mechanical and antibiotic preoperative bowel preparation can be very helpful in decreasing the overall amount of bowel distention. Also, if bowel injury occurs during the procedure, it can be laparoscopically or surgically repaired at the time.

In addition, in male patients, if a pelvic procedure is planned, it is helpful to place a Kerlex wrap around the scrotum, thereby trapping the testicles within the scrotum and compressing the scrotal skin against the testicles. The same precaution may be taken with the phallus using a separate Kerlex wrap. This will preclude the occurrence of a pneumoscrotum or pneumophallus during the procedure.

PATIENT POSITIONING

All laparoscopic procedures begin with the patient lying supine. If it is felt that arm boards will interfere with the cephalad movement of the surgeon and the assistant (see Fig. 2-1), intravenous access should be obtained via the neck, so that the patient's arms can be tucked in at the sides. However, for all other procedures, the arms can be placed on arm boards and IV access obtained antecubitally.

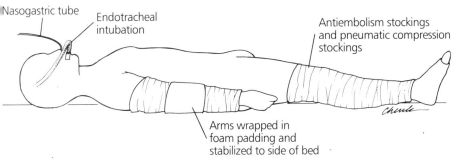

Fig. 2-1 Patient preparation.

If desired, before preparing the patient for surgery, he or she may be placed in the dorsolithotomy position. A large number of different stirrups are available; for laparoscopy it is preferable to use Allen stirrups to minimize pressure on the popliteal fossa and to distribute the weight of the leg evenly on the base of the foot. The angle of the stirrups should allow adequate access to the perineum (proper amount of abduction of the hip) while not interfering with movement of abdominal instruments (proper hip flexion) (Fig. 2-2, *A*).

Types of stirrups

In certain instances, one may benefit from use of other types of stirrups. Cane stirrups are much less cumbersome than Allen stirrups and may be easily repositioned intraoperatively. This is quite useful when performing a combined abdominal-perineal procedure. For example, during a laparoscopically assisted vaginal hysterectomy, the cane stirrups may be positioned at a 45-degree angle for the laparoscopic portion of the procedure, allowing adequate access to the abdomen. Then, to attain good perineal access, the stirrups are brought to a straight-up position for the completion of the procedure (Fig. 2-2, *B*).

The entire abdomen is prepared and draped as though a standard laparotomy were to be performed. It is helpful to include in the surgical field the phallus and testicles in the male patient and the vaginal vault in the female patient. This allows the surgeon additional manipulation of pelvic organs during the procedure, which can be beneficial during the dissection. For example, with the testicles in the surgical field, traction on either testicle can immediately delineate the location of the spermatic cord as it exits the abdomen. Similarly, in the female the

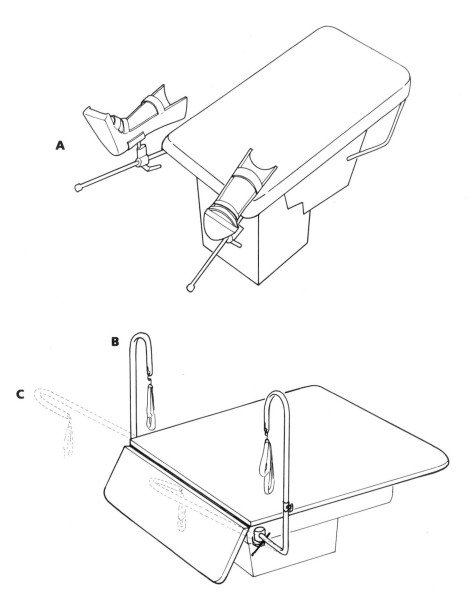

Fig. 2-2 A, Allen stirrups are useful when the dorsolithotomy position is desired. The design of these stirrups minimizes pressure on the popliteal fossa and allows one to select a variety of leg positions. **B,** Lithotomy legholders or cane stirrups, placed in the 45-degree position, allow for adequate abdominal access. **C,** Cane stirrups repositioned to 90 degrees for proper perineal access.

uterus can be manipulated to improve access to the cul-de-sac, bladder, and ovaries.

Antiembolic pneumatic compression stockings are placed on both legs. If a lengthy procedure (>2 hours) is anticipated, minidose heparin (5000 units) can be started subcutaneously 6 hours before the procedure and then given every 12 hours postoperatively until the patient is ambulatory.

Uterine manipulation is key in getting to the cul de sac, ovaries, and so on. In addition, manipulator/insufflator devices are used transvaginally so that tubal patency can be assessed.

ROOM ARRANGEMENT

For each laparoscopic procedure, the room set-up will be slightly different, depending on the patient's position. However, generally the surgeon and nurse will stand on the side of the table opposite the side of the pathologic process and the assistant will stand on the ipsilateral side of the table.

The laparoscopy cart with the television monitor and the insufflator will be at the foot of the table for pelvic procedures in which only one monitor is used (Fig. 2-3, *A*) or will be opposite the surgeon if two monitors are to be used (i.e., one on either side of the table) (Fig. 2-3, *B*). The surgeon should be able to view the television monitor and the intra-abdominal pressure, which is registered on the insufflator directly beneath the television monitor, at all times (see Fig. 2-3). Also, the monitor should be in a *direct line* with the surgical field. Hence when doing a pelvic procedure the monitor should be at the foot of the table, whereas when performing a cholecystectomy the monitor would be situated more cephalad on the right side of the table.

When using a laser, alterations in the room set-up are needed (see Fig. 2-1, *A* and *B*).

The other "lines" coming onto the table should be situated on the same side as the person who will be using that particular piece of equipment. Thus the wires to the camera, the tubing to the insufflator, and the tubing for the suction and irrigation equipment should come off the assistant's side of the table; the electrosurgical cord should come off the surgeon's side of the table. All cords and tubes should be carefully secured to the table. In addition, a "pocket" for the suction/irrigation apparatus and a pocket for the electrosurgical probe or electrosurgical scissors should be created from the drape so that these fre-

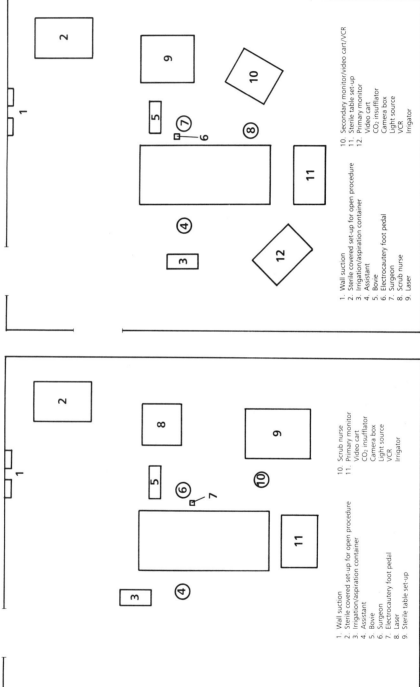

Fig. 2-3 A, Room set-up: one monitor with laser. **B,** Room set-up: two monitors with laser.

A (legend)

1. Wall suction
2. Sterile covered set-up for open procedure
3. Irrigation/aspiration container
4. Assistant
5. Bovie
6. Surgeon
7. Electrocautery foot pedal
8. Laser
9. Sterile table set-up
10. Scrub nurse
11. Primary monitor
Video cart
CO₂ insufflator
Camera box
Light source
VCR
Irrigator

B (legend)

1. Wall suction
2. Sterile covered set-up for open procedure
3. Irrigation/aspiration container
4. Assistant
5. Bovie
6. Electrocautery foot pedal
7. Surgeon
8. Scrub nurse
9. Laser
10. Secondary monitor/video cart/VCR
11. Sterile table set-up
12. Primary monitor
Video cart
CO₂ insufflator
Camera box
Light source
VCR
Irrigator

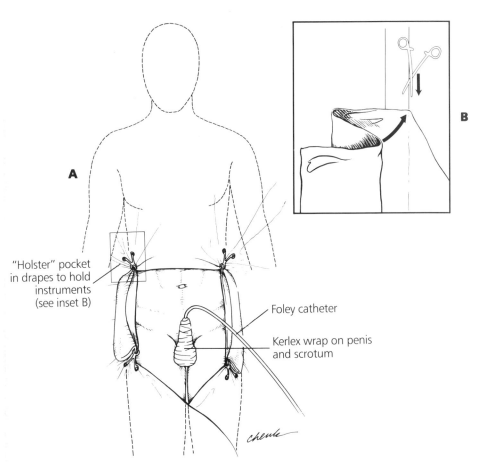

Fig. 2-4 **A,** Patient positioned and draped. **B,** "Holster" drape pocket.

quently used pieces of equipment can be properly "holstered" when not in use (Fig. 2-4, *A* and *B*).

The duties of the surgeon and assistant vary according to personal preference. Some laparoscopic surgeons prefer to operate the laparoscope and one instrument port, whereas other surgeons prefer to have the assistant operate the camera, thereby allowing them to use two instrument ports. For complex procedures the latter arrangement seems preferable, especially when dissecting delicate vascular structures.

PREOPERATIVE CHECKLIST

All instruments should be adequately tested before any laparoscopic procedure is initiated. It may be helpful to use a checklist in the operating room to ensure that all necessary equipment is present and functional (see the boxes on pp. 12-16). Specifically, the following four systems should be checked before initiating the procedure: insufflator, visualization system (camera, endoscope, monitor, light source), irrigator and aspirator unit, and electrosurgical or laser system.

The insufflator must be working properly to give an accurate measurement of intra-abdominal pressure. A *full* back-up CO_2 tank should be available in the room, and all connections between the tank and insufflator should be properly tightened to ensure that there will be no leakage.

The insufflating gas is usually supplied in size E tanks containing 1600 L of gas pressurized at 800 psi. All tanks should be checked to ensure that adequate gas pressure is available to perform the laparoscopic procedure. Gas tanks are fitted with a yoke and tubing that deliver the gas to the insufflator. The yoke is specific for each type of gas used (i.e., a CO_2 tank is fitted to a different yoke than an oxygen tank). This precludes inadvertent use of the incorrect gas for insufflation.

The insufflator is turned on, and the CO_2 tank is opened; the gauge on the insufflator should register in the green range. The flow regulator should be tested at low and high inflows and appropriate levels of flow (liters per minute) should register on the insufflator. With intra-abdominal pressure registering at 0 and with the insufflator tubing connected to the insufflator and the Veress needle (before abdominal insertion), low flow should register 1 L/min, high flow should register 2 L/min, and the intra-abdominal pressure at both settings should be ≤2 mm Hg. The cutoff intra-abdominal pressure at which CO_2 flow should cease is set by the surgeon at 15 mm Hg. When the insufflator tubing is kinked, the intra-abdominal pressure should register >15 mm Hg and the flow (i.e., liters per minute) should register 0.

Endoscopic telescopes should be inspected for damage to the lens system. The light source should be turned on and the light cable should be attached to the laparoscope. The camera should be attached to the laparoscope, focused, and white-balanced. The camera and video monitor should be turned on and a sharp picture should be seen on the monitor.

Aspiration/irrigation systems should be checked to ensure that they have been adequately cleaned and assembled. The aspirator/irrigator should be attached to the pressurized irrigating solution (1 L saline with 5000 units of heparin and 500 mg of cefazolin pressurized with a blood pump to 250 mm Hg) and to wall suction. The appropriate valves should be depressed to demonstrate that the instrument both aspirates and irrigates. If an automated aspirator/irrigator (e.g., Nezhat system) is being used, it should also be assembled, pressurized (700 mm Hg), and tested.

The electrosurgical unit should be activated. The grounding pad should be affixed to the patient. The appropriate electrosurgical *cord(s)* for the electrosurgical instruments to be used should be on the table. The foot pedal for the electrosurgical unit should be placed by the surgeon's dominant foot.

The laser should be turned on, test-fired, and then placed in the standby mode. A "laser in use" sign should be posted on the operating room door.

When a CO_2 laser is to be used it is helpful to remove the arm board and tuck the patient's arm on the side of the table where the laser will be located. This will provide space for the unit to be adequately close to the operative field. Before a procedure begins, the equipment necessary to deliver the laser beam should be available and functional. This includes either an operative laparoscope with appropriate coupling devices to deliver the laser beam parallel to the field of vision or separate guides that allow for the laser to be directed through a second operative port. The nurse or technician responsible for the laser should also ensure that a fine-focused red spot (helium-neon laser) is present before beginning the procedure. When fiberoptic lasers are used, one must make sure that the appropriate-sized fibers are in the room, as well as their ancillary equipment, which includes cleavers, strippers, irrigation/aspiration channels, and fiber diverters. Regardless of the type of laser used, the appropriate setting should be selected in advance. Appropriate safety precautions, including an active smoke evacuation system and eye protection measures, should be practiced. Hospital policies concerning laser certification should be followed, and only personnel adhering to these policies should be allowed to operate this equipment.

Finally, all operative instruments (graspers, scissors, trocars, clip applicators, and so on) need to be checked to ensure that their working components move freely and are secure. Electrosurgical instruments need to be carefully inspected to be certain that the insulation is intact along the entire shaft of the instrument and that the electrosurgical connecting cables fit properly into the instrument.

REFERENCES

1. ACOG Committee Opinion. Qualifications and privileges for performing gynecologic intra-abdominal laser therapy. No. 75, Nov 1989.
2. Keye WR. Laser Surgery in Gynecology and Obstetrics, 2nd ed. Chicago: Year Book Medical Publishers, 1990.
3. Hunt RB. Atlas of Female Infertility Surgery, 2nd ed. St. Louis: Mosby–Year Book, 1992.

CHAPTER 3

Anesthetic Considerations for Laparoscopic Surgery

Terri G. Monk and B. Craig Weldon

The ideal anesthetic technique for laparoscopy should maximize safety by reducing the risk of the cardiopulmonary complications.[1] As with all anesthetics, the technique must provide adequate amnesia, analgesia, and muscle relaxation. Because the laparoscopic approach is associated with minimal postoperative pain and a short hospital stay, the anesthetic must also allow for rapid postoperative recovery.

PATIENT PREPARATION

Preparing the patient for laparoscopic surgery presupposes a thorough understanding of the patient's medical condition, the surgical technique, and potential perioperative complications (Chapter 13). For all laparoscopic procedures, strict adherence to preoperative and intraoperative checklists will ensure optimal results (see the box on p. 25). Before any planned surgical procedure, the patient must be evaluated by an anesthesiologist. Preexisting medical conditions may significantly alter the risk of laparoscopy and must be thoroughly elucidated before an anesthetic plan is selected. After a discussion of the patient's operative risk and the anesthetic technique, informed consent is obtained.

Anesthesia for laparoscopy

Preoperative checklist

- ☐ Preoperative visit
- ☐ Informed consent
- ☐ NPO for food: 8 hours; NPO for clear liquids: >2 to 3 hours
- ☐ Consider prophylactic administration of H_2-receptor antagonist and metoclopramide
- ☐ 18-gauge (or larger) IV line
- ☐ Type and screen
- ☐ Laparotomy set-up available
- ☐ Foley bladder catheter
- ☐ Oral or nasogastric tube
- ☐ Check patient position and pad pressure points
- ☐ Compression stockings (+ / − pneumatic)
- ☐ Patient securely strapped to OR table

Monitoring checklist

- ☐ Standard intraoperative monitors (i.e., ECG, blood pressure, temperature, stethoscope)
- ☐ Pulse oximeter
- ☐ Capnometer
- ☐ Direct arterial and pulmonary artery pressure monitors in patients with severe preoperative cardiac or pulmonary problems
- ☐ Cuffed endotracheal tube if general anesthesia will be employed

---

Laparoscopic surgery is associated with an increased risk of regurgitation and aspiration of gastric contents, especially when performed on an emergency basis.[2,3] Solid food passes through the stomach at variable rates, and it is recommended that patients fast for at least 8 hours before surgery.[4] However, recent studies have shown that gastric fluid volumes are less in patients given 150 ml of water within 2 to 3 hours of induction of anesthesia when compared with patients who have fasted.[5,6] It has been suggested that the liquid bolus increases gastric peristalsis and emptying; thus small volumes of clear fluid may be permitted until 2 to 3 hours before the scheduled surgery.[4] Prophylactic administration of an H_2-receptor antagonist (e.g., cimetidine, ranitidine) can increase gastric pH. Metoclopramide, a dopamine antagonist, can also be administered preoperatively to stimulate gastric emptying and increase the tone of the lower esophageal sphincter.[7] A recent study found the combination of an H_2-receptor antagonist and metoclopramide to be the most effective pharmacologic approach for reducing risk factors for acid aspiration.[8] Therefore it is wise to administer oral ranitidine, 150 mg, in combination with oral metoclopramide, 10 mg, to patients with diseases that increase their risk for aspiration (e.g., morbid obesity, hiatal hernia, diabetic gastroparesis). These drugs are administered 2 hours before surgery with up to 150 ml of water.

During trocar insertion, perforation of a major vessel or hollow viscus can occur. The risk of significant hemorrhage strongly argues for the insertion of an 18-gauge (or larger) intravenous line, performance of type and screen assessments for blood, and a laparotomy set-up in the operating room. If a major procedure is to be performed (e.g., splenectomy, nephrectomy), a type and cross-match for 2 units is recommended. In all cases, the patient should be given the option of banking his or her own blood preoperatively.

The incidence of organ perforation can be reduced by decompression of the bladder with a Foley catheter and of the stomach with an orogastric or nasogastric tube before abdominal insufflation.

Laparoscopic procedures often require the use of the head-down position and frequent changes in the position of the operating table. To decrease the risk of peripheral neuropathy, all bony prominences should be padded, and the arms should be tucked at the patient's sides. The patient should be secured to the operating table with Velcro straps or 3-inch cloth tape at the level of the ankles, hips, and shoulders.

INTRAOPERATIVE MONITORING

Routine intraoperative monitoring for patients undergoing laparoscopic procedures consists of an electrocardiogram, a noninvasive blood pressure monitor, temperature monitor, and a stethoscope to assess breath sounds and heart tones.[9] When an anesthesia circuit is used to administer oxygen, an in-line oxygen analyzer should also be used. In addition, patients who are intubated and whose lungs are being mechanically ventilated should have continuous tidal volume and airway pressure monitoring.

Cardiopulmonary derangements are among the most common group of complications encountered during laparoscopy (see Chapter 13). This fact alone *mandates the use of pulse oximetry and capnography on all patients* undergoing general anesthesia for laparoscopic procedures. Pulse oximetry uses a light-emitting diode, placed on the finger or ear, to detect light absorbance differences between reduced hemoglobin and oxyhemoglobin.[9] This provides the anesthesiologist with a continuous, noninvasive assessment of the patient's arterial oxygen saturation. Normal values for the pulse oximeter saturation (SpO_2) are >93%. Mild hypoxia is generally considered to exist if the SpO_2 is <90%, and severe hypoxia occurs at an SpO_2 <85%.[10] If severe hypoxia is not recognized and corrected, cellular and organ dysfunction and injury may result. Pulse oximetry identifies critically low SpO_2 states as they develop and allows for intervention before cyanosis or organ dysfunction becomes clinically apparent.

Capnography is a means of monitoring the exhaled CO_2 contained in each breath. The exhaled CO_2 measured at the end of a tidal breath (end-tidal CO_2) is a close approximation of the patient's arterial CO_2 tension under most clinical situations.[11] In a normal capnogram (Fig. 3-1), the waveform resembles a mesa- or plateau-shaped structure. At the beginning of exhalation, the CO_2 tension rapidly rises and reaches a plateau level, which lasts throughout exhalation. The end-exhalation or end-tidal CO_2 value is measured at the point just before inspiration returns the CO_2 in the breathing circuit to 0. Ordinarily, the end-tidal CO_2 is 5 to 7 mm Hg lower than the $PaCO_2$ as a result of dilution of exhaled tidal volume gas with dead space gas. In general, the end-tidal CO_2 should be maintained between 30 and 40 mm Hg, which usually ensures that the $PaCO_2$ is ≤50 mm Hg.

Whenever the dead space ventilation becomes abnormally large in relation to the patient's tidal volume (e.g., in the presence of pulmonary embolus or chronic obstructive pulmonary disease), the difference between $PaCO_2$ and end-tidal CO_2 increases (i.e., enhanced dilution effect). Thus, in addition to capnography, periodic arterial blood gas sampling (i.e., every 1 to 2 hours) to determine arterial pH, $PaCO_2$, and PaO_2 may be helpful.

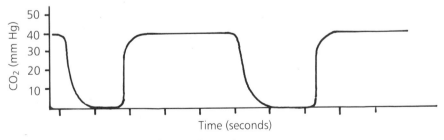

Fig. 3-1 Normal capnogram.

For an unhealthy patient undergoing a laparoscopic procedure, invasive hemodynamic monitoring is required.[12] Deciding which patients should receive invasive monitoring during laparoscopic procedures involves balancing the risks of placing and maintaining an intravascular catheter against the benefits provided by that particular monitor. Patients with severe preexisting cardiovascular or pulmonary disease who are undergoing invasive laparoscopic procedures should be considered candidates for systemic and pulmonary arterial blood pressure monitoring. However, because of the pressurized pneumoperitoneum and the use of a head-down position, one must remember that central venous and pulmonary artery pressures may not accurately reflect venous return and cardiovascular performance during laparoscopy (Chapter 13).

ANESTHETIC TECHNIQUES FOR LAPAROSCOPIC SURGERY

Laparoscopic surgery has been performed under all three major anesthetic techniques: local, regional, and general anesthesia. The choice of anesthetic technique should be based on the medical condition of the patient, the indication for the procedure, the preference of the patient, and the surgeon's needs.

Local/monitored anesthesia care

Local anesthesia may be considered for *brief* (≤60 minutes) laparoscopic procedures (e.g., diagnostic laparoscopy, tubal ligation, exploration for a cryptorchid testicle).[1,13-15] Approximately 5 ml of local anesthetic (0.5% to 1% lidocaine or 0.5% bupivacaine) is infiltrated into the skin and subcutaneous tissues at each potential trocar site. The addition of 1:200,000 epinephrine to the local anesthetic solution will approximately double the duration of infiltration anesthesia and reduce systemic absorption of local anesthetics by approximately one third.[16] Before an intra-abdominal structure is manipulated, it may be sprayed with 4 to 6 ml of anesthetic solution through the irrigator/aspirator. Care must be taken not to exceed the maximal toxic dose of the local anesthetic solution (e.g., 0.5 ml/kg of 1% lidocaine or 0.5 ml/kg of 0.5% bupivacaine).

A monitored anesthesia care (MAC) technique, in which an anesthesiologist administers additional sedative-hypnotic and analgesic medication, is often used in conjunction with local anesthesia.[15] Titration of midazolam (usual adult dose, 2.5 to 7.5 mg) and fentanyl (usual adult dose, 50 to 150 μg) is common during these procedures.[15,17] We have also used a continuous infusion of propofol (loading dose of 0.5 mg/kg intravenously followed by a maintenance infusion rate of 50 μg/kg/min) in combination with fentanyl (50 to 200 μg) to provide sedation and analgesia during these procedures.[18] With all MAC techniques, the doses of sedative-hypnotic and analgesic medications should be carefully titrated to minimize cardiorespiratory depression and permit a rapid recovery after surgery.

The advantages of a local anesthetic technique include avoidance of the risks of general anesthesia, decreased incidence of postoperative nausea and vomiting, and rapid postoperative recovery.[1] In addition, an awake, cooperative patient can alert the anesthesiologist to discomfort that may be the first sign of developing complications. However, awake patients may also experience intraoperative anxiety, respiratory compromise, abdominal pain, and shoulder pain from referred diaphragmatic irritation by the insufflating gas.[1] Thus local anesthesia or MAC techniques are best reserved for brief laparoscopic procedures that can be performed with a gentle surgical technique on cooperative patients.

Regional anesthesia

Spinal or epidural anesthesia has not gained wide acceptance for laparoscopic procedures. Many anesthesiologists believe that patients will be unable to tolerate the respiratory compromise or shoulder pain secondary to diaphragmatic irritation during abdominal insufflation.[1,19] However, Bridenbaugh and Soderstrom[20] successfully anesthetized 100 healthy women scheduled for laparoscopic tubal ligation with lumbar epidural blocks using 20 ml of 3% chloroprocaine. Surgeon and patient acceptance of the technique was high; only one patient stated that she would have preferred a general anesthetic. In addition, this technique resulted in short postanesthetic recovery periods and a low incidence (4%) of nausea and vomiting. Thus epidural anesthesia may be a safe alternative to general anesthesia in healthy patients who are undergoing relatively brief (<2 hours) laparoscopic procedures.

General anesthesia

Most therapeutic laparoscopic procedures are performed with the patient under general anesthesia. With this technique the patient experiences complete amnesia and analgesia, and the surgeon is guaranteed a quiet, relaxed patient. Both head-down positioning and increased intra-abdominal pressure predispose the patient to regurgitation and aspiration of gastric contents. Thus endotracheal intubation with a cuffed tube is recommended. During general anesthesia the patient's ventilation should be controlled to compensate for intraoperative pulmonary alterations (Chapter 13).

Major complications and morbidity are rare during laparoscopic procedures using general anesthesia. However, minor postoperative problems (nausea, vomiting, headache, myalgia, shoulder pain, dizziness) occur in most patients and appear to be related to the type of anesthetic agent used.[21-23] Dhamee et al.[21] compared halothane, enflurane, and fentanyl as supplements to nitrous oxide for general anesthesia during laparoscopy and found that postoperative nausea and vomiting were more frequent in the fentanyl-treated patients and headache was more common in patients who received a halothane anesthetic. However, a study examining postoperative complaints following anesthesia with three inhalational agents (halothane, enflurane, isoflurane) showed that the incidence of postoperative headaches was higher in patients receiving isoflurane (44%) as compared with enflurane (12%) and halothane (20%).[23] A study by De Grood et al.[24] compared postoperative recovery and side effects in patients who received total intravenous anesthesia (TIVA) with patients who received inhalational anesthesia for laparoscopic procedures. The investigators found that a TIVA technique with propofol resulted in less nausea and faster postoperative recovery as compared with an inhalational anesthetic technique with isoflurane.

Despite the differences in minor postoperative problems with the various general anesthetic techniques, there is no difference in long-term recovery. The outcome for these procedures is probably more influenced by close intraoperative monitoring and the experience of both the surgeon and anesthesiologist than the particular anesthetic technique used (see the box below).

General anesthesia recommendations

- ☐ Intubate with a cuffed endotracheal tube
- ☐ Control ventilation and adjust ventilatory patterns to compensate for intraoperative pulmonary abnormalities (goals: end-tidal CO_2 <40 mm Hg; Spo_2 ≥93%)
- ☐ Avoid prolonged intra-abdominal pressure >15 mm Hg
- ☐ Close communication between surgeon and anesthesiologist throughout the procedure

The administration of nitrous oxide during general anesthesia for laparoscopic surgery is a controversial issue. Advantages of nitrous oxide include a decreased intraoperative requirement for additional inhaled or intravenous anesthetics and a rapid induction and emergence from anesthesia. However, there are several hypothetical and actual problems with prolonged administration of nitrous oxide. Many surgeons believe that the administration of this agent makes operating conditions more difficult, because the intraoperative use of 70% to 80% nitrous oxide may increase gas volume in the bowel by 100% in 2 hours.[25] However, Taylor et al.[26] reported that the operating surgeon was unable to predict the use of nitrous oxide by assessing intraoperative bowel distention during laparoscopic cholecystectomy procedures lasting 70 to 80 minutes. It is not known whether bowel distention would become a factor in longer laparoscopic procedures or those performed in close proximity to the intestines. Other problems associated with nitrous oxide include increased incidence of postoperative nausea and vomiting and the potential for a rapidly expanding pneumothorax if an inadvertent pleurotomy occurs or an intraperitoneal explosion results if the bowel is perforated. Thus further studies are needed to determine whether the benefits of nitrous oxide administration truly outweigh its risks.

POSTOPERATIVE ANALGESIA

Near the completion of a laparoscopic procedure, postoperative pain management may be aided by intramuscular or intravenous injection of a nonsteroidal anti-inflammatory agent such as ketorolac tromethamine (Toradol). This is ideally given approximately 30 minutes before completion of the procedure. In addition, injection of a local anesthetic such as 0.25% marcaine with epinephrine into the abdominal incisions may minimize postoperative incisional discomfort.

CONCLUSION

There is no single anesthetic technique for laparoscopic surgery that is best for all patients. However, for brief diagnostic procedures, monitored anesthesia care is often sufficient, whereas for longer, more complex procedures, a general anesthetic is required.

REFERENCES

1. Fishburne JI, Keith L. Anesthesia. In Laparoscopy. Baltimore: Williams & Wilkins, 1977, pp 69-85.
2. Carlsson C, Islander G. Silent gastropharyngeal regurgitation during anesthesia. Anesth Analg 60:655-657, 1981.

3. Duffy BL. Regurgitation during pelvic laparoscopy. Br J Anaesth 51:1089-1090, 1979.
4. Stoelting RK, Miller RD. Preoperative medication. In Basics of Anesthesia. New York: Churchill Livingstone, 1989, pp 121-135.
5. Sutherland AD, Maltby JR, Sale JP, Reid CRG. The effect of preoperative oral fluid and ranitidine on gastric volume and pH. Can J Anaesth 34:117-121, 1987.
6. Maltby RJ, Koehli N, Shaffer EA. Gastric fluid volume, pH, and emptying in elective inpatients: Influences of narcotic-atropine premedication, oral fluid, and ranitidine. Can J Anaesth 35:562-566, 1988.
7. Stoelting RK. Gastric antacids, stimulants, and antiemetics. In Pharmacology and Physiology in Anesthetic Practice. Philadelphia: JB Lippincott, 1987, pp 433-443.
8. O'Sullivan G, Sear JW, Bullingham RES, Carrie LES. The effect of magnesium trisilicate mixture, metoclopramide, and ranitidine on gastric pH, volume and serum gastrin. Anaesthesia 40:246-253, 1985.
9. Stoelting RK, Miller RD. Monitoring. In Basics of Anesthesia. New York: Churchill Livingstone, 1989, pp 211-227.
10. Yelderman M. Pulse oximetry. In Monitoring in Anesthesia and Critical Care Medicine. New York: Churchill Livingstone, 1990, pp 417-427.
11. Gravenstein JS, Paulus PA, Hayes TJ. Carbon dioxide and monitoring. In Capnography in Clinical Practice. Boston: Butterworth, 1989, pp 3-10.
12. Rao TK. Cardiac monitoring for the noncardiac surgical patient. Semin Anesth 2:241-250, 1983.
13. Brown DR, Fishburne JI, Roberson VO, Hulka JF. Ventilatory and blood gas changes during laparoscopy with local anesthesia. Am J Obstet Gynecol 124:741-745, 1976.
14. Alexander GD, Goldruth M, Brown EM, Smiler BG. Outpatient laparoscopic sterilization under local anesthesia. Am J Obstet Gynecol 116:1065-1068, 1973.
15. Wall RT, Gelmann EP, Hahn MB, Jelenich SE. Monitored anesthesia care for laparoscopies in oncology patients. Anesthesiology Rev 18:43-48, 1991.
16. Stoelting RK. Local anesthetics. In Pharmacology and Physiology in Anesthetic Practice. Philadelphia: JB Lippincott, 1987, pp 148-168.
17. Zelcer J, White PF. Monitored anesthesia care. In Anesthesia. New York: Churchill Livingstone, 1990, pp 1321-1334.
18. Monk TG, Bouré B, White PF, Meretyk S, Clayman RV. Comparison of intravenous sedative-analgesic techniques for outpatient immersion lithotripsy. Anesth Analg 72:616-621, 1991.
19. Mulroy MF. Regional anesthesia: When, why, why not? Probl Anesth 2:82-92, 1988.
20. Bridenbaugh LD, Soderstrom RM. Lumbar epidural block anesthesia for outpatient laparoscopy. J Reprod Med 23:85-86, 1979.
21. Dhamee MS, Gandhi SK, Calleen KM, Kalbfleisch JH. Morbidity after outpatient anesthesia: A comparison of different endotracheal anesthetic techniques for laparoscopy. Anesthesiology 57:A375, 1982.
22. Collins KM, Docherty PW, Plantevin OM. Postoperative morbidity following gynecological outpatient laparoscopy. Anaesthesia 39:819-822, 1984.
23. Tracey JA, Holland JC, Unger L. Morbidity in minor gynecological surgery: A comparison of halothane, enflurane, and isoflurane. Br J Anaesth 54:1213-1215, 1982.
24. De Grood PMRM, Harbers JBM, van Egmond J, Crul JP. Anaesthesia for laparoscopy: A comparison of five techniques including propofol, etomidate, thiopentone, and isoflurane. Anaesthesia 42:815-823, 1987.

25. Eger EI, Saidman LJ. Hazards of nitrous oxide anesthesia in bowel obstruction and pneumothorax. Anesthesiology 26:61-66, 1965.
26. Taylor E, Feinstein R, Soper N, White PF. Effect of nitrous oxide on surgical conditions during laparoscopic cholecystectomy. Anesthesiology 75:541-543, 1991.
27. Neuman GG, Sidebotham G, Negoianni E, Bernstein J, Kopman AF, Hicks RG, West ST, Haring L. Laparoscopy explosion hazards with nitrous oxide. Anesthesiology 78:875-879, 1993.
28. Helvacioglu A, Weis R. Operative laparoscopy and postoperative pain relief. Fertil Steril 57(3):548-552, 1992.

CHAPTER 4

Establishing the Pneumoperitoneum

Louis R. Kavoussi and Nathaniel J. Soper

In establishing a pneumoperitoneum, there are two essential pieces of equipment: the insufflator and the Veress needle.

INSUFFLATOR

When the insufflator is turned on, the CO_2 pressure should register in the green, indicating sufficient tank pressure. The CO_2 cylinder should be checked to be certain that it contains sufficient gas for the completion of the procedure. If there is any doubt, a new CO_2 container should be brought into the OR. *A spare tank of CO_2 should always be available in the room.*

The sterile insufflation tubing is connected to the insufflator. Next, the insufflator is turned to high flow (>6 L/min); at this point with the insufflator tubing not yet connected to a Veress needle or laparoscopy sheath, the intra-abdominal pressure indicator should register 0 (Fig. 4-1). Next, the insufflator flow should be lowered to 1 L/min flow. The tubing is kinked; the intra-abdominal pressure indicator should rapidly rise to 30 mm Hg and the registered flow of CO_2 should cease (Fig. 4-2). It is essential to the performance of safe laparoscopy that the pressure/flow shutoff mechanism be operational.

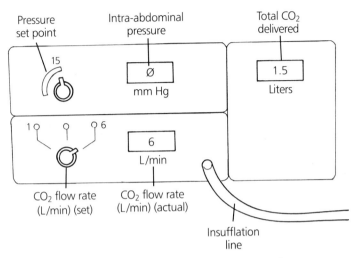

Fig. 4-1 Insufflator testing. With insufflator tubing open (i.e., not connected to Veress needle) and flow rate set at 6 L/min, the intra-abdominal pressure reading obtained through the open insufflation line should be 0 mm Hg.

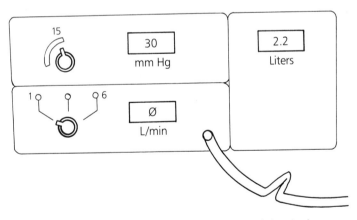

Fig. 4-2 With the insufflation tubing kinked, the intra-abdominal pressure should rapidly rise (e.g., 30 mm Hg), thereby exceeding the preset 15 mm Hg pressure set point. The flow of CO_2 should immediately cease (0 L/min).

The flow regulator should be tested at low and high inflow. With the insufflator tubing connected to the insufflator and the Veress needle (before abdominal insertion), low flow should register 1 L/min and high flow should register 2 L/min; the intra-abdominal pressure at both settings should be ≤3 mm Hg. A pressure reading >3 mm indicates a blockage in the hub or shaft of the Veress needle; if this occurs, the needle should be replaced. Maximal flow through a Veress needle is only 2 L/min, regardless of the insufflator setting, because of the 14-gauge size of the needle. However, when an open cannula is placed, it can immediately accommodate the maximum flow rate of most insufflators (i.e., >6 L/min).

VERESS NEEDLE

Either a disposable or nondisposable Veress needle may be used. The former is a one-piece plastic design (external diameter, 2 mm; 14 gauge; length, 70 or 120 mm), whereas the latter is made of metal and can be disassembled. The needle is checked by flushing saline from a syringe through it to ensure its patency. With a disposable needle, the tip of the needle should be occluded and the fluid pushed into the needle under moderate pressure to be certain there is no leakage from the plastic hub. If there is a leak, a new needle should be obtained. Likewise, on nondisposable Veress needles, all seals must be checked and the "screws" tightened.

Next, the blunt tip of the Veress needle is pushed against the handle of a knife or a solid, flat surface to be certain that the blunt tip will retract easily (Fig. 4-3, A) and will spring forward rapidly and smoothly (Fig. 4-3, B). A red indicator in the hub of the disposable needle can be seen to move upward as the tip retracts (see Fig. 4-3). The tip of the needle must not be damaged during this process.

PNEUMOPERITONEUM

The supine patient is placed in a 10- to 20-degree head-down position. In an abdomen that has not been previously operated, the site of entry is at the level of the superior (abdominal procedures) or inferior (gynecologic pelvic procedures) border of the umbilical ring or directly through the umbilicus (obese patient) (Fig. 4-4). The inferior margin of the umbilicus can be immobilized by pinching the superior border of the umbilicus between the thumb and forefinger of the nondominant hand and rolling the superior margin of the umbilicus in a cephalad direction. Alternatively, in the asleep patient, a small towel clip can be placed on either side of the upper margin of the umbilicus; this makes it a bit easier to stabilize the umbilicus and lift it upward. Next, a hook

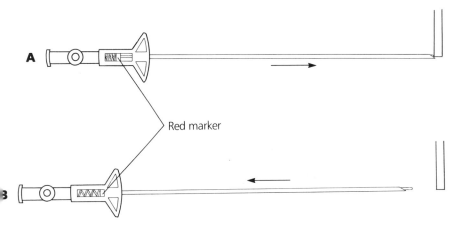

Fig. 4-3 Testing retractable tip of disposable Veress needle. **A,** Blunt tip retracts as it contacts resistance (e.g., a knife handle). **B,** When the needle is pulled away from the point of resistance, the blunt tip springs forward in front of the sharp edge of the needle.

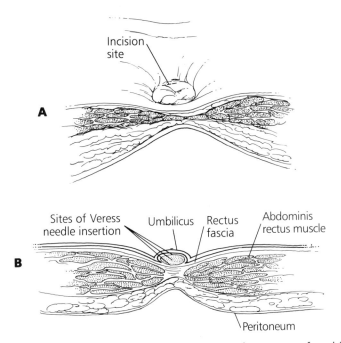

Fig. 4-4 A, Site of Veress needle insertion at superior crease of umbilicus; stab incision has been made. **B,** Transverse oblique section at superior crease of umbilicus; the peritoneum is closer to the skin at the umbilicus and is more densely adherent to the umbilicus than at any other site along the abdominal wall.

(No. 12) blade can be used to make a tiny stab incision in the midline of the superior or inferior margin or center of the umbilicus. With the dominant hand, the *shaft* (not the hub) of the Veress needle is grasped like a dart and gently passed into the wound—either at a 45-degree caudal angle to the abdominal wall (in the asthenic or minimally obese patient) or perpendicular to the abdominal wall in the markedly obese patient. Resistance followed by a give will be felt at two points: as the needle meets and traverses the fascia and then as it touches and traverses the peritoneum (Fig. 4-5). As the needle enters the peritoneal cavity, a distinct click can often be heard as the blunt tip portion of the Veress needle springs forward into the peritoneal cavity.

Next, a 10 cc syringe with 5 cc of saline is connected to the Veress needle. The first step is to *aspirate* to assess whether any blood or bowel contents (yellow fluid) enter the barrel of the syringe. The second step is to instill the 5 cc of saline; it should flow into the abdominal cavity without resistance. The third step is to aspirate again. If the peritoneal cavity has truly been reached, no saline should return. Fourth, the stopcock is closed as the syringe is disconnected from the Veress needle; the stopcock is then opened and any fluid left in the hub of the syringe should rapidly fall into the abdominal cavity, especially if the abdominal wall is elevated slightly with the towel clips. If free flow is not present, the needle is either not in the cavity, or it is adjacent to a structure. Fifth, if the needle truly lies in the peritoneal cavity, the surgeon should be able to advance it 1 to 2 cm deeper into the peritoneal cavity without encountering any resistance. Specifically, the tip indicator or the hub of the needle should show no sign that the blunt tip of the needle is retracting, thereby indicating the absence of fascial or peritoneal resistance.

It is crucial to be cognizant of the anatomic landmarks when placing the needle, and once the needle is in place it should be stabilized during insufflation. Movements of the needle from side to side as well as back and forth should be minimized in view of the potential complications associated with Veress needle insertion and CO_2 insufflation.

Once the surgeon is certain the tip of the Veress needle lies in the peritoneal cavity, the insufflation line can be connected to the Veress needle. The flow of CO_2 should be turned to 1 L/min, and the indicator on the machine for total CO_2 infused should be reset to 0. The pressure in the abdomen during initial insufflation should always register less than 10 mm Hg (after subtracting any pressure noted when the needle was tested by itself with the insufflator) (Fig. 4-6).

If high pressures are noted or if there is no flow because the 15 mm Hg limit has been reached, the surgeon can gently rotate the needle to

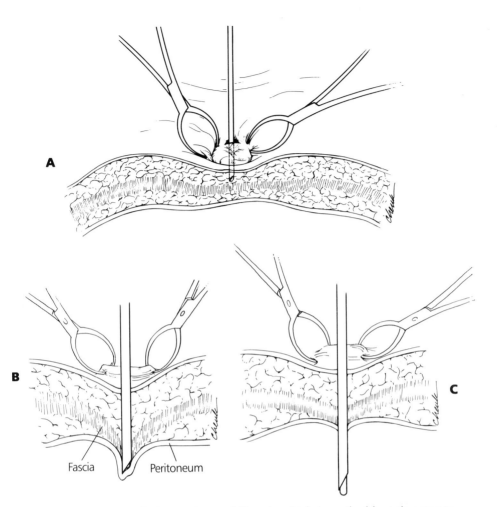

Fig. 4-5 A, Veress needle inserted at umbilicus (sagittal view; the blunt tip retracts as it encounters the fascia of the linea alba). **B,** As the sharp edge of the needle traverses the fascia, the blunt tip springs forward into the properitoneal space and then retracts a second time as it encounters the peritoneum. **C,** Blunt tip springs forward as Veress needle passes across the peritoneum to enter the abdominal cavity.

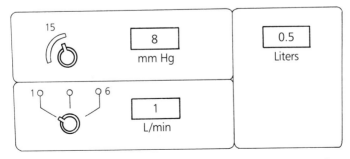

Fig. 4-6 Initial insufflation readings: proper inflow at beginning of CO_2–Veress needle insufflation.

assess whether the opening in the shaft of the needle is resting on the abdominal wall, omentum, or the bowel; the inflow hole on the shaft of the needle is on the same side of the needle as the stopcock. If the abdominal pressure remains high (i.e., needle in adhesion, omentum, or properitoneal space), then the needle should be withdrawn before 200 ml of CO_2 are instilled; another pass of the Veress needle can then be made. If necessary, this process can be repeated several times until the surgeon is certain that the needle resides within the peritoneal cavity. Insufflation should not be continued if the surgeon is uncertain about the appropriate intraperitoneal location of the tip of the Veress needle; multiple passes with the Veress needle are not problematic, provided the error is not compounded by insufflating the "wrong" space.

One of the first signs that the Veress needle lies truly in the abdomen is loss of the dullness to percussion over the liver during early insufflation. When the needle is correctly placed, the peritoneum should effectively seal off the needle; if CO_2 bubbles out along the needle's shaft during insufflation, one must suspect a properitoneal location of the needle tip. Likewise, during insufflation a previously unoperated abdomen should appear to expand symmetrically, and there should be loss of the normal sharp contour of the costal margin.

The patient's pulse and blood pressure are monitored closely during the early phase of insufflation to ensure that a vagal reaction does not occur. If the pulse falls precipitously, the CO_2 is allowed to escape, atropine is administered, and insufflation is reinstituted slowly after a normal heart rate has returned.

After 1 L of CO_2 is insufflated, the flow of CO_2 should be increased to ≥ 6 L/min (Fig. 4-7). (Even though the flow on the machine is set at 6 L/min, the maximal flow achievable through a 14-gauge Veress needle is only 2.5 L/min.) Once the 15 mm Hg limit is reached, the actual flow of CO_2 will cease. At this point approximately 3 to 6 L of CO_2 should have been instilled into the abdomen (Fig. 4-8). When percussed, the abdomen should sound as though one is thumping a ripe watermelon.

Alternative methods of obtaining a pneumoperitoneum

In selected female patients, alternative methods of establishing a pneumoperitoneum are useful. These include passage of the Veress needle through the posterior fornix (cul de sac) or transuterine (transfundal) needle passage. These methods may prove useful when conventional attempts are unsuccessful or contraindicated, or as a primary procedure in obese patients.

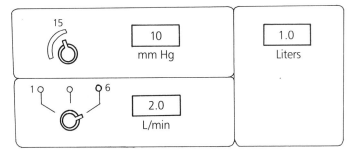

Fig. 4-7 After 1 L is insufflated, the set flow is increased to the highest rate.

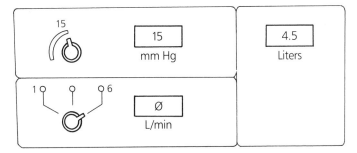

Fig. 4-8 At 15 mm Hg intra-abdominal pressure, 3 to 6 L of CO_2 will usually have been insufflated; the registered flow should then fall to 0.

Placement of the Veress needle via the posterior fornix has been demonstrated to be safe as well as effective. The needle must be placed in the midline about 1.75 cm behind the junction of the vaginal vault and the smooth epithelium of the posterior cervical lip. It is helpful to have a long Veress needle; however, one should be careful not to advance the needle beyond a depth of 3 cm. This method should not be attempted in individuals with an abnormal cul de sac (Fig. 4-9, A).

Transuterine insertion of the Veress needle is a useful alternative route in obese patients. This method is often contraindicated if uterine fibroids are present and should be used cautiously in patients that may have periuterine adhesions. Active pelvic infections and pregnancy are clear contraindications. Patients are placed in the head-down position and the cervix is grasped with a tenaculum. The uterine position and

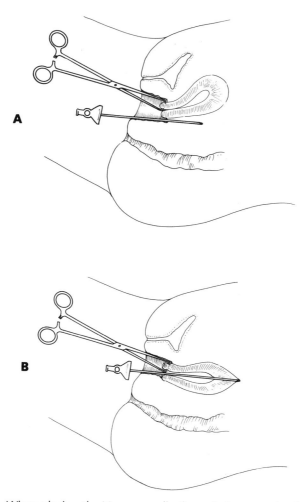

Fig. 4-9 A, When placing the Veress needle through the posterior fornix, one must stay in the midline and not advance the needle beyond 3 cm. **B,** Transfundal needle insertion is done while stabilizing the cervix with a tenaculum. After sounding the uterus, the needle is passed transuterine directed away from the sacral curve, rectosigmoid, and large vessels. The needle is removed under direct visualization after the laparoscope has been placed.

size are evaluated with uterine ultrasonography, and the Veress needle is grasped by the collar and directed away from the sacral curve, rectosigmoid, and large vessels. The needle is slowly inserted; the spring release occurs when the tip of the needle has entered the peritoneal cavity (Fig. 4-9, *B*). After the location has been verified and the pneumoperitoneum established, the primary trocar is placed in the conventional fashion. The Veress needle is then removed under direct visualization. If dye insufflation is desired, the uterine hole may be occluded with a blunt probe.

Alternative to a pneumoperitoneum

Laparoscopic surgery may be suitably accomplished with no pneumoperitoneum whatsoever using abdominal wall lift techniques. These methods have been designed to eliminate the undesirable physiologic effects of *any* gas instilled under *any* pressure. These devices "lift the roof" of the abdomen from the underlying viscera to establish exposure and a working space. Devices reported to date include polyethylene sling devices, subcutaneous tunneled wires, or T- or L-shaped devices placed under the abdominal wall (Fig. 4-10). Further studies will be necessary to establish that these techniques are safe, cost effective, and do not add to the pain and morbidity of the laparoscopic procedure.

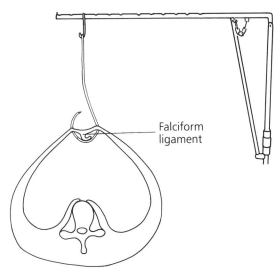

Falciform ligament

Fig. 4-10 Abdominal wall lift technique.

TROUBLESHOOTING

Problem: Machine registers low pressure in the CO_2 tank.
Solution: Obtain a new tank of CO_2.

Problem: High pressure registered when CO_2 is insufflated in the Veress needle before the needle has been placed in the body.
Solution: Get a new Veress needle or clear the channel of the 14-gauge Veress needle by washing it with saline and passing a 3 Fr guidewire through it.

Problem: Aspiration of yellow fluid.
Solution: Needle is probably in bowel. Remove the needle and repuncture the abdomen. After successful insertion of the laparoscope, closely inspect abdominal viscera for a significant injury.

Problem: Aspirate reveals blood.
Solution: Remove the needle and repuncture the abdomen. Once access to the abdomen has been achieved, a full examination of the retroperitoneum to look for an expanding retroperitoneal hematoma is mandatory. Likewise, if there are any hemodynamic changes, this should alert the surgeon to the possibility of a significant vascular injury.

Problem: Aspirate reveals saline.
Solution: The needle is probably in the properitoneal space. The needle needs to be advanced deeper to pierce the peritoneum.

Problem: High pressures (e.g., 10 to 15 mm Hg) are obtained during insufflation at 1 L/min.
Solution: The needle probably is in the properitoneal space, omentum, or directly adjacent to the viscera. Rotate the needle 90 degrees. If high pressure persists, remove the needle and repuncture the abdomen.

Problem: Subcutaneous crepitance.
Solution: Replace the needle because it is probably in the subcutaneous space.

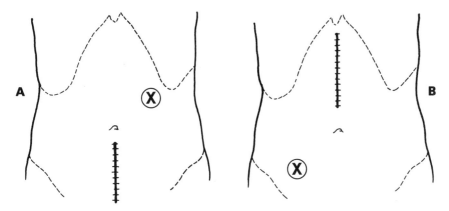

Fig. 4-11 A and **B,** Optional trocar sites in previously operated abdomen. (NB: Consider open-cannula technique.)

Problem: Previously operated abdomen with a midline incision.

Solution: For a *lower* midline incision, place Veress needle in the upper left quadrant of the abdomen just lateral to the rectus sheath. Realize that the properitoneal space here is more easily insufflated than at the umbilicus and that the needle may therefore need to be passed more deeply into the abdomen in order to enter the peritoneal cavity. The right upper quadrant should be avoided because of the size of the liver and the presence of the falciform ligament (Fig. 4-11, *A*). For an upper midline incision, place the needle in the right lower quadrant, since in older patients there are usually sigmoid adhesions in the left lower quadrant (Fig. 4-11, *B*).

Problem: Previously operated abdomen with a solitary incision in an upper or lower abdominal quadrant.

Solution: Pass the Veress needle in the opposite abdominal quadrant just lateral to the rectus muscle. Avoid the right upper abdominal quadrant if at all possible because of the size of the liver and the presence of the falciform ligament (see Fig. 4-11). Also avoid the left lower quadrant because of sigmoid adhesions that may be present despite the patient's not recalling any history of diverticulitis (Fig. 4-12).

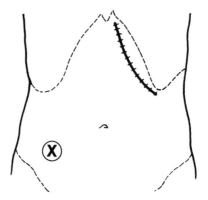

Fig. 4-12 Veress needle replacement in the event of a prior left upper quadrant incision. (NB: Consider open-cannula technique.)

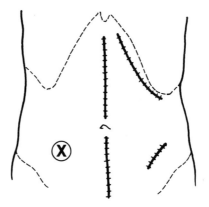

Fig. 4-13 Veress needle placement in the event of multiple prior abdominal incisions. (NB: Consider open-cannula technique.)

Problem: Previously operated abdomen in multiple quadrants.
Solution: Use a Veress needle or open cannula in an area farthest removed from existing abdominal scars (Fig. 4-13) (see Chapter 5). If the open cannula is to be used, an open cut-down technique is recommended. When in doubt, the open-cannula technique remains the safest method for entering the abdomen.

Problem: Suspected CO_2 embolus.

Solution: Desufflate abdomen. Immediately place patient in right-side-up, head-down position. If a CVP line is present, attempt to aspirate CO_2 from the right side of the heart by advancing the CVP line until it is in the right side of the heart. If a pulmonary catheter is in place, try to aspirate CO_2 through the catheter (see Chapter 13).

REFERENCES

1. Soper NJ. Laparoscopic cholecystectomy. Curr Probl Surg 28:585-655, 1991.
2. Banting S, Shimi S, Velpen GV, Cuschieri A. Abdominal wall lift: Low pressure pneumoperitoneum in laparoscopic surgery. Surg Endosc 7:57-59, 1993.
3. Leighton TA, Bongard FS, Liu SY, Lee TS, Klein SR. Comparative cardiopulmonary effects of helium and carbon dioxide pneumoperitoneum. Surg Forum 42:485-487, 1991.
4. Neely MR, McWilliams R, Makhlouf HA. Laparoscopy: Routine pneumoperitoneum via the posterior fornix. Obstet Gynecol 45:459-460, 1975.
5. Wolfe WM, Pasic R. Instruments and methods. Obstet Gynecol 75:456-457, 1990.
6. Morgan HR. Laparoscopy: Induction of pneumoperitoneum via transfundal puncture. Obstet Gynecol 54:260-261, 1979.

CHAPTER 5

Abdominal Access: Initial Trocar Placement

Howard N. Winfield

The laparoscopic trocar is the means through which abdominal access is secured. As with the Veress needle, the placement of the first trocar is usually a "blind" procedure with significant potential complications. Thus a thorough understanding of the construction of the trocar and the method for its proper insertion are extremely important.

The primary trocar is the first trocar to be placed after obtaining a pneumoperitoneum. For therapeutic procedures, this trocar is usually ≥ 10 mm (sheath size) and has a sidearm for CO_2 insufflation; for diagnostic procedures, a 5 mm sheath with a sidearm can be used.

There are a variety of trocar sizes and types available. A list of the various trocars available is provided in Appendix A. All trocars have two common components: a sharp *obturator* to facilitate entry into the abdominal cavity (Fig. 5-1, *A*) and a *sheath* through which the obturator passes (Fig. 5-1, *B* and *C*). The sheath contains a valve or membrane through which instruments may be introduced without the loss of CO_2 from the abdomen. Also, the sheath may or may not have a side port for insufflation of CO_2.

REUSABLE TROCARS

Trocars are either reusable or disposable. *Reusable* trocars usually are equipped with a conical or pyramidal pointed obturator in which a small channel may be drilled for the length of the shaft (see Fig. 5-1, A-C). This channel allows for the audible release (i.e., hiss) of CO_2 as soon as the gas-filled abdomen is entered, thereby signaling that the trocar has entered the abdomen to a sufficient depth for delivery of the sheath. The valve in these trocars is usually of a trumpet type. The valve should be checked before inserting the trocar to ensure that it can be easily depressed (i.e., opened) and that it spontaneously returns to its resting (i.e., closed) position. Also, with reusable trocars the obturator should be resharpened after a maximum of 16 uses.

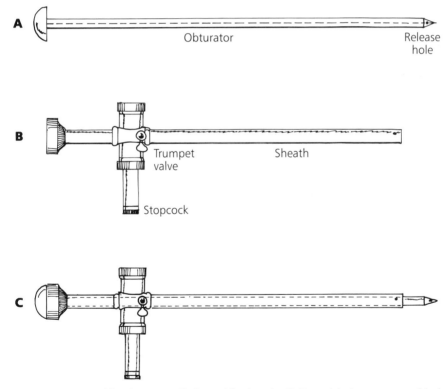

Fig. 5-1 **A,** Reusable obturator. **B,** Reusable sheath. **C,** Reusable trocar, assembled.

DISPOSABLE TROCARS

Disposable trocars may have a conical or, more commonly, pyramidal pointed obturator (Fig. 5-2, *A*) but without a channel drilled the length of the shaft. To appreciate entry into the abdomen, the sidearm stopcock is turned to the open position; a rush of CO_2 from the sidearm indicates that the sheath is well situated within the gas-filled abdomen (Fig. 5-2, *B*). The valve mechanism is either a flap valve or a soft plastic membrane (Fig. 5-2, *B* and *C*).

Two other features available on some of the disposable trocars are a safety shield and a retention mechanism. The safety shield is a spring-loaded, blunt plastic outer covering that retracts as the trocar meets the

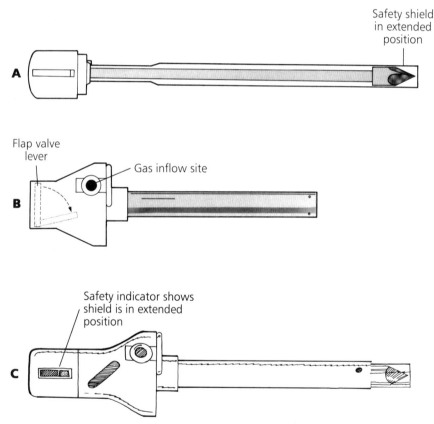

Fig. 5-2 A, Disposable obturator. **B,** Disposable sheath. **C,** Disposable trocar, assembled.

resistance of the abdominal wall (Fig. 5-3, *A*) and automatically slides over the sharp tip of the obturator when the trocar enters the resistance-free, gas-filled abdomen. Once released, the safety shield locks in its forward position, thereby covering the sharp tip of the obturator and decreasing the risk of inadvertent injury to underlying viscera (Fig. 5-3, *B*).

Obviously the shield must be retracted during passage of the trocar. The shield is usually inactivated by pushing the obturator firmly into the sheath of the trocar and firmly grasping the obturator and sheath so they form a complete unit. As the firmly held trocar is introduced into the skin site, the safety shield encounters the resistance of the abdominal wall and begins to retract, thereby exposing the abdominal wall to the sharp point of the obturator; at the time it retracts, a single click is heard. If the operator inadvertently relaxes the pressure that holds the obturator firmly within the sheath, there will be a second audible click, signalling that the safety shield has descended over the tip of the obturator and has *locked* in place. When this occurs, the cylindrical, blunt safety shield is now locked in its forward position, thereby covering the sharp tip of the obturator and precluding deeper passage of the trocar into the abdominal wall. Accordingly, the trocar

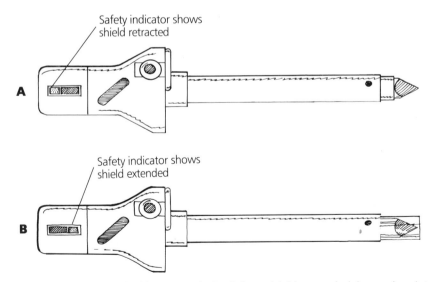

Fig. 5-3 A, Safety shield retracted. **B,** Safety shield extended beyond point of obturator.

must be "rearmed" by again firmly grasping it so that the obturator is seated tightly against the sheath. The trocars equipped with a safety shield also have an indicator on the obturator that clearly shows when the safety shield is activated (i.e., locked over the obturator's tip) or deactivated (i.e., capable of spontaneous retraction during passage of the trocar into the abdomen) (see Fig. 5-3, A and B).

The safety shield is not failsafe and does *not* preclude injury to underlying viscera. If the incision used for introduction of the trocar is of insufficient size, the safety shield may hang up at the skin level and thus be unable to spring back into position after the sharp trocar tip has entered the abdominal cavity. This occurrence is usually signified by excessive resistance met while trying to introduce the trocar through the abdominal wall. The problem is remedied by lengthening the incision to a size large enough to accept the full diameter of the safety shield on the sheath.

The *retention* feature on some disposable trocars consists of a ribbed or grooved area on the outside of the sheath (Fig. 5-4, A and B). The ribbed area may be molded into the sheath or may be a separate collar that fits around the sheath (i.e., a ribbed collar and a locking nut). In the latter case, once the sheath is positioned deep within the abdominal cavity, the collar is screwed down over the sheath until it traverses the abdominal wall. The sheath can then be retracted through the collar until it extends only 2 cm into the abdomen; the locking nut on top of the collar is tightened, thereby fixing the collar to the sheath. The entire assembly is now secure within the abdominal wall (Fig. 5-5, A and B). Alternative retention features include an inflatable balloon and a four-wing Malecot arrangement.

There is one potentially dangerous combination of an outer collar and the sheath: specifically, *a metal sheath should never be used in combination with an outer plastic collar.* This assembly can result in electrosurgical complications from conductance, since the plastic collar precludes abdominal wall dissipation of any current conducted to the metal sheath. This buildup of current on the sheath can potentially damage any viscera or bowel that is in contact with the sheath.

TROCAR INSERTION

In an unoperated abdomen the initial trocar is usually passed at the inferior (for pelvic procedures) or superior (for upper abdominal procedures) crease of the umbilicus. This location is chosen because the abdominal wall is thinnest at this level. At the level of the umbilicus,

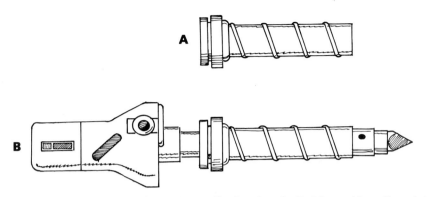

Fig. 5-4 A, Disposable self-retaining collar for sheath. **B,** Disposable self-retaining collar placed onto sheath of trocar.

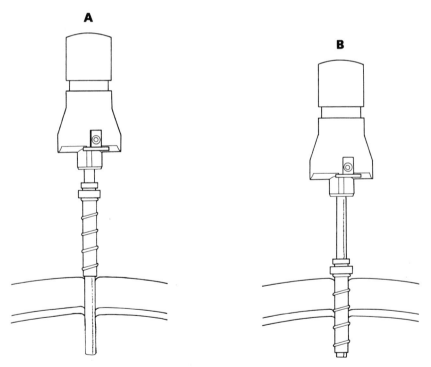

Fig. 5-5 A, After trocar sheath is positioned, the self-retaining collar, **B,** is screwed through the abdominal wall.

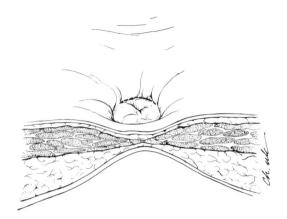

Fig. 5-6 Umbilical incision along superior crease.

the properitoneal layer, which lies between the linea alba and the peritoneum, is the thinnest (Fig. 5-6). The postoperative scar at this site is cosmetically acceptable; it becomes indistinguishable from the umbilicus itself. Also, there are no significant blood vessels that traverse this area.

There are only a few potential contraindications to an umbilical entry: a midline incision, portal hypertension and a recanalized umbilical vein, and umbilical abnormalities. The last problems from an umbilical entry arise from an unrecognized urachal cyst, urachal sinus, or umbilical hernia. The skin at the umbilical crease (superior or inferior) is incised circumferentially or vertically until the incision is long enough to accept the *full* circumference of the ≥10 mm sheath (and extended safety shield) assembly of the trocar (see Fig. 5-6). A hook blade (No. 12) is helpful, because with it a more exact incision can be made. The skin incision can be spread with a Kelly clamp in a cephalocaudal direction; this helps the incision to assume a more rounded configuration, thereby conforming to the round shape of the trocar and may displace the underlying fat, thereby possibly reducing any bleeding from the subcutaneous fat as it is traversed by the sharp tip of the trocar (Fig. 5-7). Next, with a No. 15 stab blade, a small nick is made in the rectus fascia (linea alba); this will facilitate passage of the obturator through the midline fascia. (NB: Be careful to nick just the fascia; if the peritoneum is incised during this maneuver, the pneumoperitoneum will begin to leak.)

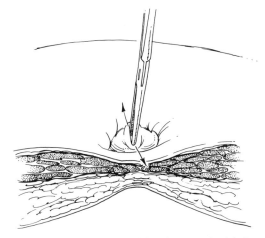

Fig. 5-7 Superior umbilical incision is spread with forceps.

In preparation for passage of the initial trocar, the patient can be placed either supine or in a 10- to 30-degree head-down position.

Alternatively, if one prefers to lift the abdominal wall manually (Fig. 5-8), then the abdominal pressure should be kept at only 10 to 15 mm Hg. The intra-abdominal pressure is transiently increased to 20 to 25 mm Hg, thus further distending the peritoneal cavity and pushing the peritoneum more firmly against the overlying abdominal wall. This maneuver, in theory, facilitates the passage of the trocar across the peritoneum and increases the volume of the pneumoperitoneum by 30%.

The surgeon holds the fully assembled ≥10 mm trocar in the palm of the dominant hand; the outer aspect of the obturator is firmly secured against the thenar eminence and pushed into the sheath. The index or middle finger is extended down the shaft of the sheath to act as a brake; this will prevent the trocar from being suddenly advanced too deep into the abdomen. The sidearm of the trocar is turned to the open position. The nondominant hand may be used to grasp and raise the anterior abdominal wall directly beneath the umbilicus (see Fig. 5-8). Alternatively, a large towel clip may be placed on either side of the umbilical incision; the nondominant hand is then used to hold up the towel clip nearer the surgeon while the assistant grasps and raises the other towel clip slightly upward, thereby stabilizing the abdominal wall

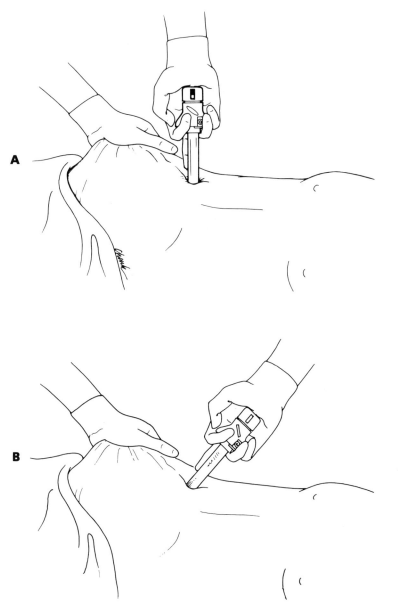

Fig. 5-8 A and **B,** Middle finger is braced along the shaft of the trocar as the trocar is pushed through the abdominal wall; the abdominal wall is stabilized with the nondominant hand.

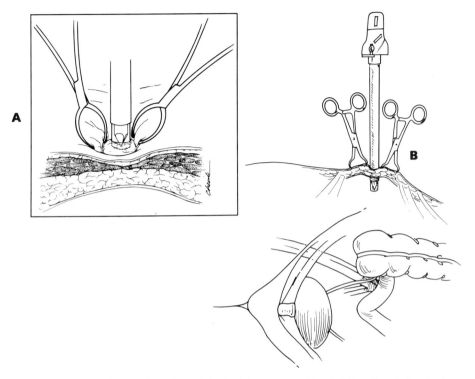

Fig. 5-9 A, Towel clips at the edge of the incision are used to stabilize the abdominal wall during trocar insertion. **B,** By stabilizing the abdominal wall, the distance between the abdominal wall and the bowel is maintained during trocar passage.

(Fig. 5-9, *A* and *B*). No effort is made to elevate the abdominal wall; the purpose of the towel clips is to prevent the posterior movement of the abdominal wall as the trocar is passed.

The angle of the midline insertion of the ≥10 mm trocar is initially perpendicular (Fig. 5-9, *A*). A steady downward minimally twisting force is applied to the trocar unit (Fig. 5-10). Care must be taken not to move the trocar back and forth, or else the tissue will be stretched from side to side and the chances of CO_2 leaking along the sheath will be increased.

Once the tip of the obturator is through the skin incision and subcutaneous fat, the trocar handle is tilted cephalad to a 60- to 70-degree

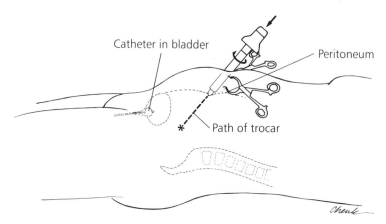

Fig. 5-10 After perpendicular passage through the umbilical incision, the trocar is directed toward an imaginary point midway between the sacral promontory and the bladder.

angle; thus the tip of the obturator is directed toward an imaginary point midway between the sacral promontory and the bladder (see Fig. 5-10). This point lies well below the bifurcation of the aorta and vena cava. In an obese patient, the trocar insertion should be directly perpendicular, since the umbilicus is displaced caudally and the perpendicular route is the shortest path into the abdominal cavity.

The surgeon must not relax the grip on the trocar; if this occurs, the obturator will become disengaged from the sheath and a click will be heard. The click indicates that the safety shield has moved to its forward position and is now locked, thereby precluding passage of the trocar, since the sharp tip of the obturator is now covered by the blunt plastic safety shield. If at any time during passage of the trocar a click is heard, the trocar must be rearmed by reseating the obturator within its sheath so that the safety shield will properly retract, thereby exposing the tissue of the abdominal wall to the sharp tip of the obturator.

As the peritoneal cavity is entered, the operator should appreciate an audible click as the safety shield springs forward and locks in front of the tip of the obturator. As the obturator is withdrawn, escaping CO_2 creates a "whooshing" sound as it rapidly flows out of the opened side port of the trocar. The sidearm port is now closed. The trocar is advanced

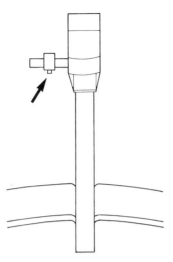

Fig. 5-11 Sidearm *(arrow)* is closed and the sheath is advanced deeper into the peritoneal cavity.

1 to 2 cm deeper into the abdomen and the obturator is removed (Fig. 5-11).

Alternatively, if a nondisposable trocar is used, the first indication of entry into the peritoneal cavity will be a loss of resistance as the fascia and peritoneum are transversed, followed by a similar "whooshing" rush of CO_2 from the small hole drilled along the length of the obturator. Next, the obturator is retracted slightly (so only the dull tip of the sheath protrudes into the abdominal cavity). The sheath is advanced 1 to 2 cm into the abdomen and the obturator is removed. The trap door, flap, or trumpet valve of the sheath automatically seals, thereby precluding loss of any of the intra-abdominal CO_2.

Direct trocar insertion

Placement of the primary trocar without prior pneumoperitoneum has been widely used in some centers. Large series have been reported that have shown this technique to be safe and efficient. This procedure is contraindicated in patients suspected of having significant adhesions of the anterior abdominal wall.

After the anesthetized patient is properly positioned, a 1 cm skin incision is made and the tissues spread to the level of the fascia (Fig. 5-12, *A* and *B*). The abdominal wall is then elevated by grasping with an open 4 × 4 gauze sponge on each side of the midline. The 10 mm trocar and sleeve is then directed toward the pelvic hollow in a slow, controlled fashion. The loss of resistance, similar to when a pneumoperitoneum is present, signals an intra-abdominal location. The trocar is removed (Fig. 5-12, *C*) and the position confirmed by visualization with the laparoscope. When the proper location is ensured, insufflation is begun.

Proponents of this technique point out that many of the complications of laparoscopy are related to improper insufflation or needle placement. It is quicker than conventional methods, and inserting a trocar through a nondistended abdominal wall makes it much easier to feel individual tissue layers and avoids the high force–low control sometimes required with a taut abdominal wall. Properitoneal insufflation should not occur with this technique.

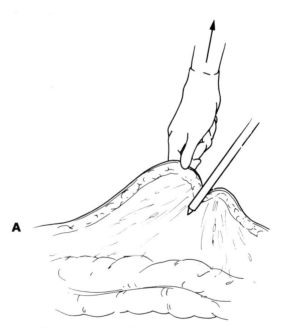

A

Fig. 5-12 A 1 cm skin incision is made in the umbilicus. **A,** The abdominal wall is elevated and the trocar and sheath are directed toward the pelvic hollow.

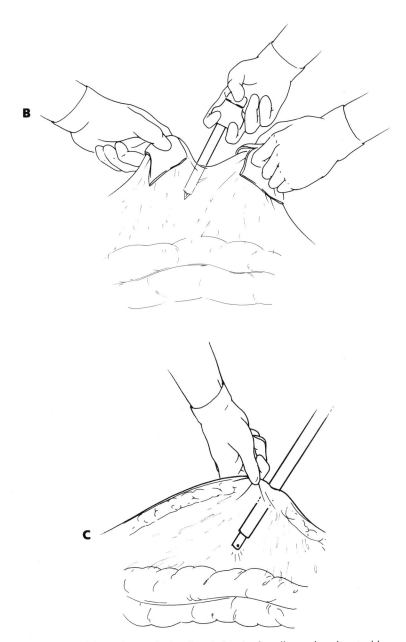

Fig. 5-12, cont'd B, Alternatively, the abdominal wall may be elevated by grasping each side with an open 4 × 4 gauze pad. **C,** The trocar is removed and the laparoscope inserted. Insufflation is begun only after proper location is ensured.

OPEN CANNULA

The open (e.g., Hasson) cannula provides the surgeon with an alternative, extremely safe method to enter the abdomen, especially in a patient who has undergone multiple intra-abdominal procedures. In these patients in particular, the blind insertion of a trocar would be fraught with the potential for injury to the bowel or omentum. The open cannula may also be used routinely in all patients for placement of the initial umbilical trocar, depending on the surgeon's preference. The open cannula consists of three pieces: a cone-shaped sleeve, a metal or plastic sheath with a trumpet or flap valve, and a blunt-tipped obturator (Fig. 5-13). On the sheath or on the cone-shaped sleeve, there are two struts for affixing two fascial sutures. The cone-shaped sleeve can be moved up and down the sheath until it is properly positioned; it can then be tightly affixed to the sheath. The two fascial sutures are then wrapped tightly around the struts, thereby firmly seating the cone-shaped sleeve into the fasciotomy and peritoneotomy. This creates an effective seal so the pneumoperitoneum will be maintained.

An incision is made in the quadrant of the abdomen farthest away from any of the preexisting abdominal scars or in the infraumbilical skin crease if there has been no prior midline surgery (see Chapter 4). For example, the incision for the open cannula is made just lateral to the rectus muscle in the upper left abdominal quadrant if a midline abdominal incision is present. If there is no midline abdominal incision, a periumbilical incision can be made. An incision approximately 2 to 3 cm long is made in a transverse direction. The subcutaneous tissue is dissected with scissors, and the underlying fascia is identified and in-

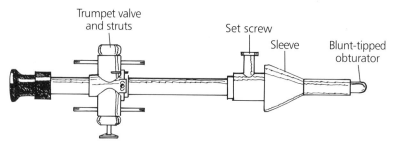

Trumpet valve
and struts

Set screw

Sleeve

Blunt-tipped
obturator

Fig. 5-13 Open (Hasson) cannula: reusable type.

cised (Fig. 5-14, *A*). The properitoneal fat is gently swept off the peritoneum in a very limited area. The peritoneum is grasped between hemostats and opened sharply (Fig. 5-14, *B*). This incision should be just long enough to admit the surgeon's index finger. Entry into the abdominal cavity is confirmed visually and by passing an index finger through the incision to palpate the inside of the abdomen. Digital palpation ensures the absence of adhesions in the vicinity of the incision. An 0-absorbable suture is placed on either side of the fascial incision.

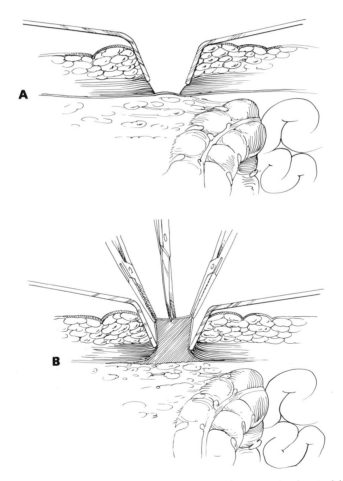

Fig. 5-14 A, Retractors expose peritoneum. **B,** Peritoneum is elevated by clamps and sharply incised.

The completely assembled open cannula is inserted through the peritoneotomy with the blunt tip of the obturator protruding. Once the obturator is well within the abdominal cavity, the conical collar of the open cannula is advanced down the sheath until it is firmly seated in the peritoneal cavity. The collar is secured to the sheath with the set screw. The two separate fascial sutures are secured to the struts on the sheath or collar of the open cannula, thereby fixing the cannula in place (Fig. 5-15). The CO_2 line is connected to the sidearm port of the cannula,

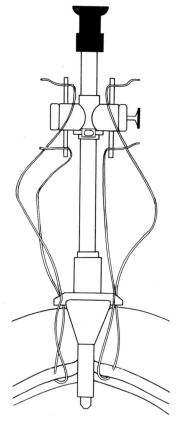

Fig. 5-15 Two fascial sutures are secured to the struts on the sheath of the non-disposable open cannula. The cone-shaped sleeve is then pushed firmly into the fasciotomy and peritoneotomy and the set screw is tightened, thereby fixing the sleeve to the sheath of the open cannula. The sutures are now wound tightly around the struts on the sheath, thereby securing the sheath in place and sealing the fasciotomy and peritoneotomy.

and the blunt-tipped obturator is withdrawn; a pneumoperitoneum is established with the insufflator set at high flow. The intra-abdominal pressure is raised to 15 mm Hg.

Once one gains facility in the open-cannula technique, one can create a pneumoperitoneum as fast as or faster than can be done with Veress needle and "blind" trocar passage. Indeed, this is the safest way to establish a pneumoperitoneum.

If an open cannula is not available, two concentric purse-string mono-filament sutures may be placed in the midline fascia and an incision made in the center of the pursestrings into the free peritoneal cavity. Both sutures are kept long and the tails of each suture are passed through a 3 cm segment of a red rubber catheter, thereby creating two modified Rummel tourniquets. A standard laparoscopic sheath (with the sharp-tipped trocar removed) is then placed and the purse-string sutures are cinched against the sheath and secured by placing a clamp on the red rubber Robinson catheter. At the conclusion of the operation, the fascia is closed by simply tying the sutures to each other.

TROUBLESHOOTING

Problem: Unable to advance trocar into abdomen.
Solution: The entire circumference of the plastic safety shield must enter the skin before the trocar is pushed into the peritoneal cavity (see Fig. 5-9, A). Check the skin site. If the skin incision is too small, the plastic safety shield will hang up on the skin as it retracts, thereby preventing the forward advance of the trocar. (NB: The unshielded sharp tip of the trocar may be exposed to the peritoneal contents at this time, thereby causing injury to the bowel or any underlying viscera.)

Problem: Trocar injury: large vessel (e.g., iliac, aorta, inferior vena cava): early diagnosis.
Recognition: As soon as the obturator is removed, if the injury is to an *artery*, blood will immediately fill the sidearm; intra-abdominal pressure will immediately rise above 15 mm Hg and CO_2 flow will cease. As the obturator is pulled from the sheath, blood will escape from the sheath under significant pressure (Fig. 5-16, A-C). If the injury is to a major *vein* (e.g., iliac vein), as the obturator is withdrawn, blood may be seen to exit the sheath. A more ominous situation is the possibility of a CO_2 *embolus* and hypotension, since given the low venous pressure (10 mm Hg), CO_2 may be pumped into the vein.

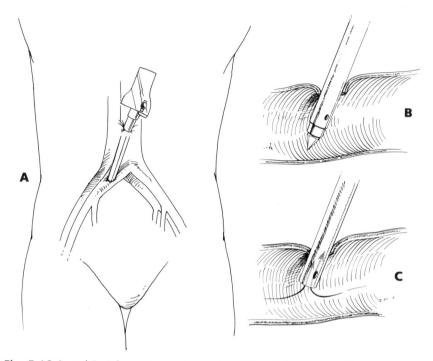

Fig. 5-16 A and **B,** Primary trocar has entered the right common iliac artery. **C,** As the obturator is withdrawn, blood fills the sheath and momentarily shoots out of the flap valve.

Solution: Open laparotomy and repair. If the injury is recognized at this point in the procedure, the sheath should be left in the vessel, thereby tamponading it. A midline incision is then made and the abdomen is widely entered. Vascular control is gained along the vessel above and below the point of sheath entry; the sheath is removed and the injury repaired. (For treatment of a CO_2 embolus, see Chapter 4 Troubleshooting.)

REFERENCES

1. Kaali SG, Barad DH. Incidence of bowel injury due to dense adhesions at the sight of direct trocar insertion. J Repro Med 37:617-618, 1992.
2. Jarrett JC. Laparoscopy: Direct trocar insertion without pneumoperitoneum. Obstet Gynecol 75:725-727, 1990.
3. Nezhat FR, Silfen SL, Evans D, Nezhat C. Comparison of direct insertion of disposable and standard reusable laparoscopic trocars and previous pneumoperitoneum with Veress needle. Obstet Gynecol 78:148-150, 1991.

CHAPTER 6

Laparoscopic Examination of the Abdomen and Pelvis

Ralph V. Clayman

Abdominal Inspection
Troubleshooting

Laparoscopes are designed in two basic configurations—end-viewing (0-degree) and oblique-viewing (angled view of 30 degrees or 45 degrees). End-viewing laparoscopes adequately visualize most areas of the abdomen, and their manipulation is easily learned. The oblique-viewing laparoscopes are slightly more difficult to use while maintaining visual orientation; however, they provide a better view of recesses within the abdominal cavity and of the anterior abdominal wall.

Before placement of the endoscope, the insufflator tubing is connected to the side port of the ≥10 mm sheath, and the intraperitoneal pressure is raised to 15 mm Hg. There are *five* steps in setting up the 10 mm laparoscope before passage into the body. First, the light source is turned on, and the light cable is connected to the endoscope. Second, the camera is locked onto the endoscope so that the image is properly oriented (i.e., up-down and left-right; "true"). Third, the camera image on the television screen is brought into sharp focus by focusing on the threads of a white gauze pad. Fourth, with the endoscope still focused on the *white* gauze pad, the camera "white-balance" button is pressed to correct the color sensitivity. Fifth, the shaft of the endoscope is prewarmed by swathing it with warm saline; the tip of the endoscope is then treated with an antifogging solution (see Appendix A).

If there is an 11 mm or a 12 mm primary sheath, a 10.5 mm reducer is applied to the sheath. Next, the 10 mm laparoscope is introduced into the abdominal cavity.

ABDOMINAL INSPECTION

Confirmation of correct positioning of the endoscope sheath within the abdominal cavity occurs with the identification of underlying loops of intestine. The retroperitoneum immediately posterior to the entry site is examined for the presence of a hematoma. The bowel underlying the point of entry is inspected for any signs of injury. Likewise, there should be no blood dripping down from the sheath; if this occurs, an abdominal wall vessel has probably been injured during trocar passage. If need be, this can be occluded after placement of a second ≥10 mm trocar. However, this bleeding is rarely of any hemodynamic significance and usually ceases of its own accord within a few minutes.

A systematic examination of the abdomen is performed. The laparoscope is directed caudally and the *lower* abdomen is inspected. The midline bladder is identified in the pelvis along with the umbilically directed, broad-based urachus (Fig. 6-1). Next, the paired prominent medial umbilical ligaments (i.e., obliterated umbilical arteries) are noted as they course from the lateral aspects of the bladder toward the umbilicus. In male patients the spermatic cord is seen as it enters the internal inguinal ring (see Fig. 6-1). Both groin areas are inspected for the presence of an inguinal hernia. In female patients the uterus, ovaries, and fallopian tubes are visualized along with the round ligament (Fig. 6-2). The inferior epigastric vessels indent the anterior abdominal wall just medial to the internal inguinal ring and lateral to the medial umbilical ligament. The lateral-lying colon is noted. On the right side, the cecum and appendix are seen.

The *upper* abdomen is then inspected. The liver, gallbladder, and stomach are viewed. The spleen is not generally visible unless the patient is in a head-up position and rotated to the right. If the spleen is readily visible with the patient supine, it is probably pathologically enlarged. The omentum and small bowel are examined for any evidence of injury from the passage of the Veress needle or the primary trocar.

If the omentum cannot be properly seen and if there is blood dripping down onto the field from the ≥10 mm sheath, then it is possible that a leaf of omentum or bowel was traversed on entry into the abdomen. Confirmation of this problem requires that a second trocar be placed; into this trocar an endoscope (5 or 10 mm, depending on the size of the second trocar) is introduced, and the point of entry of the initial trocar into the abdomen is inspected (see Chapter 7).

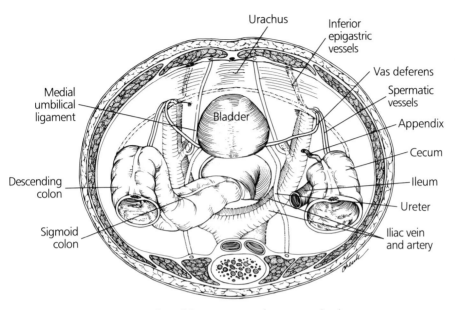

Fig. 6-1 Male pelvic anatomy—laparoscopic view.

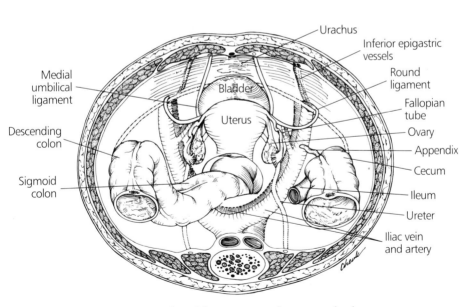

Fig. 6-2 Female pelvic anatomy—laparoscopic view.

TROUBLESHOOTING

Problem: The pneumoperitoneum pressure appears to be changing rapidly.

Solution: This probably means that there is fluid in the line and should be of no concern to the operator, provided that the pressure is ≤15 mm Hg.

Problem: Only fat is seen, and there *is* abdominal wall crepitance.

Solution: The laparoscope is probably in the subcutaneous space. The trapped CO_2 is evacuated (Fig. 6-3), and the laparoscope is withdrawn. The Veress needle is now passed through a small skin incision at the opposite border of the initial umbilical point of entry or via the left upper quadrant just lateral to the rectus muscle.

Problem: Only fat is seen, yet there *is no* abdominal wall crepitance.

Solution: The tip of the endoscope is probably through the abdominal fascia and lying in the properitoneal space. Again, the CO_2 is evacuated, but the sheath is not withdrawn. A pneumoperitoneum is obtained by inserting the Veress needle via a new midline skin incision lying 2 to 3 inches below the original skin incision. The tip of the Veress needle is passed directly in front of the tip of the laparoscope. In this case the progress of the needle across the properitoneal space and into the peritoneal cavity is visually monitored with the laparoscope (Fig. 6-4).

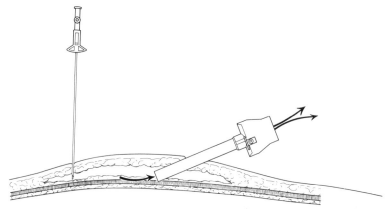

Fig. 6-3 The sheath is in the subcutaneous space; as much gas as possible is allowed to escape before reinserting the Veress needle.

Problem: Grainy-appearing fat is seen without any intervening spaces. There *is no* abdominal wall crepitance (Fig. 6-5, *A*).

Solution: The laparoscope is probably in the omentum (Fig. 6-5, *B*), and as such the endoscope should be slowly withdrawn until the abdominal cavity is seen. The surgeon should carefully inspect the omentum for any bleeding; this site should be carefully electrocoagulated before proceeding.

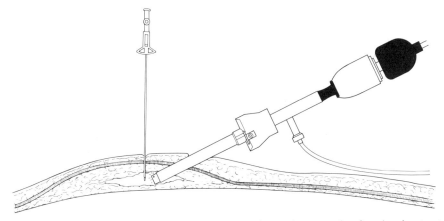

Fig. 6-4 Passage of Veress needle, under endoscopic control, after inadvertent properitoneal insufflation.

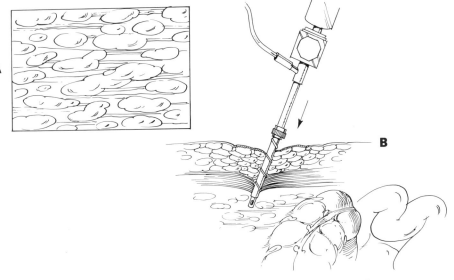

Fig. 6-5 A, View with laparoscope in omentum. **B,** Laparoscope in omentum.

Problem: Fogging.

Solution:

- Use warm water to bathe the shaft of the endoscope. In this regard a heating pad or hot plate on the back table is useful to maintain a ready supply of warm water.
- An additional sterile endoscope can be kept on the back table in the heating pan to replace an endoscope that is fogging.
- Use an antifog solution (see Appendix A); this can be applied to the tip of the endoscope before its insertion into the abdominal cavity.
- Also, fogging can be reduced or eliminated at times by gently touching the undersurface of the abdominal wall (not the bowel) with the tip of the endoscope (i.e., abdominal wipe maneuver).
- Use a cotton swab or Q-tip to wipe any blood or fluid off the top of the sheath's flap valve so it will not smear the lens of the endoscope as it is passed into the sheath. The Q-tip can also be used to swab out the inside of the sheath.
- Connect the insufflator tubing to one of the accessory sheaths; occasionally, the flow of cool CO_2 across the endoscope's lens may induce fogging.

Problem: Initial sheath pulled *partially* out of the abdomen (Fig. 6-6, *A*). There is a half-moon appearance to the peritoneotomy as the overlying fat begins to fall into the opening in the peritoneum (Fig. 6-6, *B*). In this situation, significant subcutaneous emphysema will occur and the pneumoperitoneum will decrease to the point that the surgeon will be unable to see inside the abdomen.

Solution: Under endoscopic control, maneuver the laparoscope back into the patient's abdominal cavity, then advance the sheath over the laparoscope.

Problem: Initial ≥10 mm sheath is pulled completely from the abdomen.

Solution: Place a finger over the skin incision site. Backload the ≥10 mm sheath onto the 10 mm laparoscope. Under endoscopic control advance the laparoscope back into the abdomen. Advance the laparoscope deep into the abdomen. Slide the ≥10 mm sheath over the laparoscope. If the ≥10 mm sheath cannot be visually replaced, the abdomen is reentered with a ≥10 mm trocar through the initial skin incision site.

Problem: Incorrect color scheme on monitor.

Solution: Pull the laparoscope from the abdomen and repeat the white-balancing procedure using a *clean white* gauze pad.

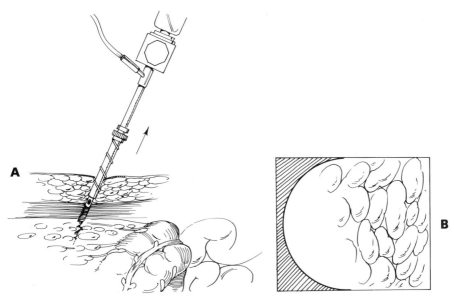

Fig. 6-6 A, Initial sheath pulled partially out of the abdomen. **B,** Laparoscopic view; note half-moon appearance of the peritoneotomy.

Problem: Air leak around the endoscope.
Solution: To create an airtight seal, a 10.5 mm reducer must be affixed to the 11 or 12 mm sheath before passage of the 10 mm laparoscope.

Problem: Air leak around the sheath.
Solution:
- Secure two 0-monofilament absorbable purse-string sutures in the skin and fascia around the sheath (Fig. 6-7, A-C). Cut the needle from the suture but do not tie the suture. Instead, cut a 2- to 3-inch section from an 8 Fr red rubber Robinson catheter and pass it over the two ends of the suture. Cinch the catheter section against the skin and secure it in place by affixing a mosquito clamp onto the tails of the suture as they exit the section of catheter. (At the end of the procedure, release the mosquito clamp, remove the section of catheter, and pull out the two sutures.)
- Wrap ¼-inch petrolatum gauze around the sheath and secure it with a separate stitch to the skin and the sheath, thereby better sealing the sheath-skin interface.
- Set CO_2 inflow at its maximal rate.

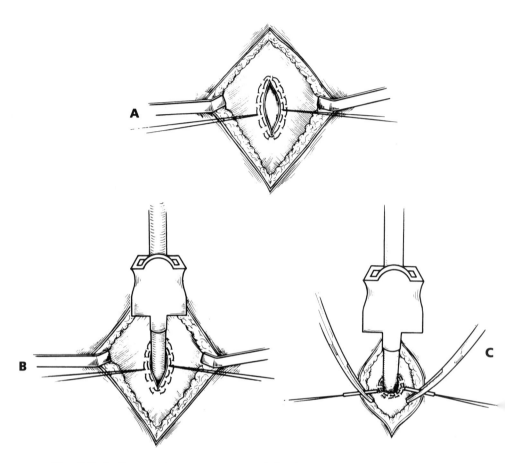

Fig. 6-7 A, Purse-string sutures around fasciotomy. **B,** Trocar inserted through fasciotomy. **C,** Purse-string sutures are tightened around the sheath of the trocar by clamping the rubber-shod portion of the suture. This will help to seal off the CO_2 leak.

Problem: Image upside down.
Solution: Camera must be locked in a *true* orientation. Rotating the 0-degree laparoscope will not affect the orientation; only by turning the camera can the field be altered. To prevent inadvertent changes in orientation, the assistant should be instructed to hold the camera, not the shaft of the laparoscope (Fig. 6-8). *WAKE UP!*

    If an oblique-viewing (e.g., 30-degree) laparoscope is being used, the endoscope and camera must both be correctly aligned (i.e., "true"). The camera must always be maintained in a "true" upright position for video orientation. The viewing lens of the oblique lap-

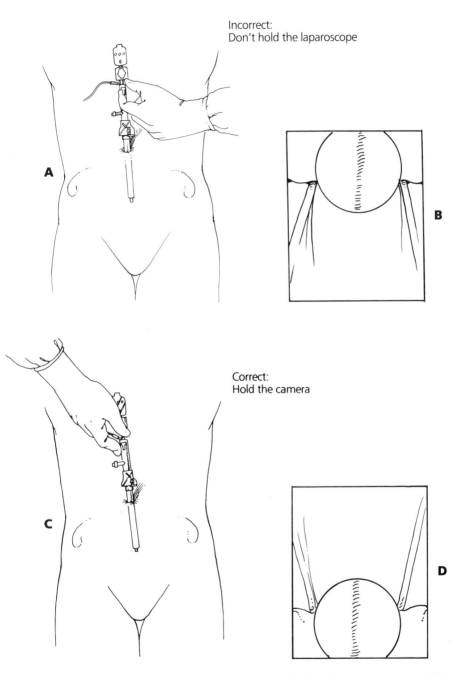

Incorrect:
Don't hold the laparoscope

A

B

Correct:
Hold the camera

C

D

Fig. 6-8 A, Camera is turned upside down on a 0-degree laparoscope. **B,** Upside-down image of bladder, medial umbilical ligaments. **C,** Camera righted. **D,** Correct ("true") image.   *Continued.*

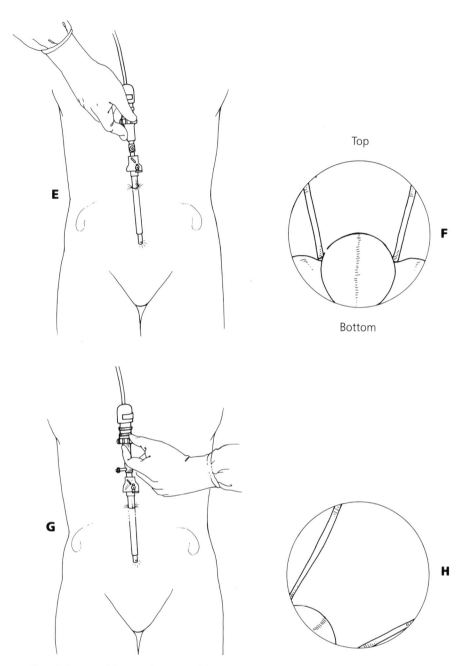

Fig. 6-8, cont'd E, When an oblique-viewing laparoscope is used, the assistant must hold the camera and endoscope so the light post points to the ceiling and neither it nor the camera can rotate. In this arrangement, a view of the abdominal contents is obtained. If the camera's position is maintained and the light post is rotated 180 degrees, then a clean view of the undersurface of the abdominal wall is seen on the television monitor **(F). G,** If the camera is rotated off alignment with the endoscope, this changes the laparoscopic image accordingly **(H).**

aroscope is angled away from the light post of the laparoscope. The field of view may be changed by rotating the laparoscope while maintaining the position of the endoscopic camera. Depending on the desired viewpoint, the endoscope may look "up" at the abdominal wall (i.e., light post down) or "down" at the posterior abdomen (i.e., light post up). This is the preferred orientation for most general exploratory surveys, because it reproduces the surgeon's viewpoint of open laparotomy. With an angled laparoscope, the assistant must be even more vigilant and endeavor to prevent any rotation of the endoscope or the camera. To do this the camera can be held in its "true" orientation and the light post can be secured with the index finger of the same hand (Fig. 6-8, *E*).

Problem: Omental insufflation.
Solution: Recognition of gaseous distention and air bubbles within the omentum requires no action. However, if there is bleeding from the omentum, electrocoagulation is necessary. This is best done after first placing two or more sheaths for passage of the irrigator and an electrosurgical forceps. The bleeding site is secured with the forceps and then electrocoagulated. The carbon dioxide within the omentum will be resorbed rapidly.

Problem: Bowel serosal insufflation.
Solution: Air bubbles in bowel serosa; no action (Fig 6-9).

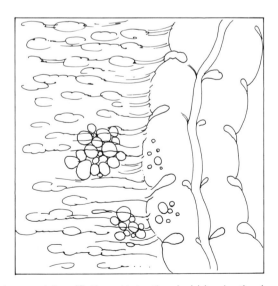

Fig. 6-9 Bowel serosal insufflation. Note tiny bubbles in the bowel serosa and mesentery.

Problem: Trocar injury: bowel, one-wall puncture.

Recognition: The red rugae of the inside of the bowel wall are appreciated. No other intra-abdominal organs are seen (Fig. 6-10, A).

Solution: By pulling back the sheath and laparoscope, the hole in the bowel can be identified (Fig. 6-10, B). This can be immediately oversewn either laparoscopically, after placement of two or more additional trocars, or by a laparotomy.

Problem: Trocar injury: large vessel (e.g., iliac, aorta, inferior vena cava).

Recognition: Hemorrhage may either be immediately apparent because of a blood-filled abdomen or the surgeon may note a "swelling" of the retroperitoneal space. As blood fills the retroperitoneum, there will be a marked decrease in the space available to work within the abdomen. Despite the adequate intra-abdominal pressure, it will

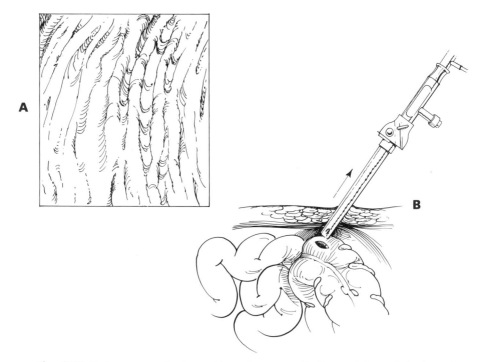

Fig. 6-10 **A,** Laparoscopic view of bowel mucosa. **B,** Trocar injury of the bowel— one-wall puncture is appreciated as the endoscope and sheath are slowly retracted.

seem as though the abdomen is no longer distended sufficiently. Vascular collapse rapidly ensues.

Solution: Open laparotomy and repair.

- The surgeon should be aware that in most individuals, directly beneath the umbilicus lies the aortic bifurcation or right common iliac vessels. Only in an obese patient does the umbilicus lie well below these major vascular structures. A trocar injury, if recognized early (i.e., before the trocar is withdrawn from the vessels), can be rapidly approached through a midline incision. *By leaving the trocar in the vessel, tamponade can be achieved.*

- If the vascular injury is noted after removal of the trocar, rapid entry into the abdomen and vascular control are essential. In this case the pneumoperitoneum is immediately evacuated and the laparoscopic sheath is swung up to the midline of the abdomen. In one motion, by cutting down directly onto the entire length of the laparoscope sheath, the surgeon enters the abdomen. A stick sponge is placed directly on the injured vessel, thereby compressing it. Vascular repair can then be undertaken after the patient has been appropriately resuscitated. For this repair the immediate aid and advice of a vascular surgeon are desirable.

  NB: The occurrence of this problem may be reduced by (1) placing the patient in a 10- to 30-degree head-down position before inserting the trocar, (2) transiently increasing intra-abdominal pressure to 20 to 25 mm Hg just before trocar insertion, and (3) directing the trocar so it is pointed at 45 degrees toward the pelvis, thereby avoiding the major pelvic vascular structures.

Problem: Trocar injury: bladder.

Recognition: The interior of the bladder is noted with its smooth urothelium (Fig. 6-11) and urethral catheter. Gas or blood is noted in the bladder drainage bag. The laparoscope is withdrawn. The site of the perforation can be located by instilling 100 to 250 cc of a saline solution mixed with indigo-carmine (10 ml indigo-carmine in 1000 cc saline) through the urethral catheter.

Solution: Place a 12 mm secondary trocar in the lower abdomen, just lateral to the rectus sheath on the same side as the bladder injury; place a 10 mm trocar in a similar position on the contralateral side. Grasp the bladder on either side of the puncture and then close the puncture site with a laparoscopic suture or gastrointestinal anastomosis (GIA) stapler (i.e., use a "tissue" load).

If this is not feasible, an open repair is recommended since the

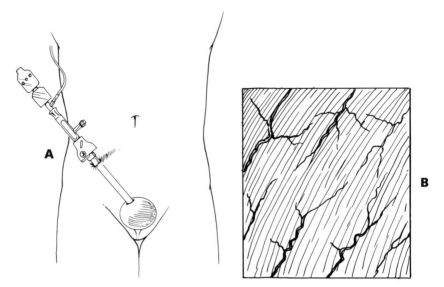

Fig. 6-11 A, Trocar injury—bladder perforation. **B,** Laparoscopic view of bladder mucosa.

bladder injury is *intraperitoneal.* In either case flexible cystoscopy should be done to identify the ipsilateral ureteral orifice. If the injury is close to the ureter, a guidewire can be passed up the ureter at this time and an external stent can be secured. Likewise, the security of the closure is tested by reinstilling the indigo-carmine/saline solution via the cystoscope or a urethral catheter.

NB: At the inception of each laparoscopic procedure, the bladder should be completely drained by properly placing a Foley urethral catheter. Also, the anesthetist should be instructed to notify the surgeon if blood-stained urine or gas collects in the drainage bag at any time during the procedure.

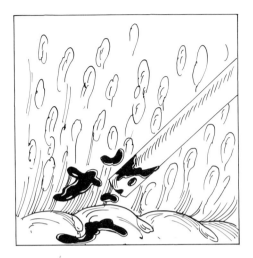

Fig. 6-12 Blood noted on bowel and bowel mesentery; the endoscopist can see drops of blood as they fall from the laparoscope. The site of bleeding is alongside the sheath where it traverses the abdominal wall.

Problem: Blood on bowel and omentum.

Recognition: If there is no visible injury to the bowel or omentum, then the blood is probably coming from the trocar site. In this case, it is dripping off the sheath. If it drips onto the endoscope, it will cover the lens and blur the image on the monitor (Fig. 6-12).

Solution: A second trocar will need to be placed so that the site of the initial trocar placement can be inspected. (See Chapter 7, Primary trocar site inspection, p. 88.) If the bleeding appears to be significant, the injured abdominal vessel can be occluded with a transabdominal suture tied over a bolster. (See Fig. 7-11 in Chapter 7, Troubleshooting, p. 97).

Secondary Trocar Placement

Ralph V. Clayman

To perform laparoscopic surgery, an additional two to five trocars must be placed to act as conduits for the surgical instruments. These additional trocars are ≥5 mm; they may lack a safety shield or insufflation sidearm and may have only a simple membrane to act as a valve. They are inserted under direct endoscopic monitoring.

SITE SELECTION

The site of placement of these additional trocars depends on the type of procedure to be performed. However, the secondary trocars must be arrayed so that they are not too close to each other; if placed too near one another, the ability to maneuver instruments within each individual sheath becomes limited as the tops of the sheaths (i.e., extracorporeal valved end) begin to interfere with each other on the abdominal surface. Also, the surgeon will experience problems in moving the instruments within the abdomen, because sheaths in close proximity will strike on one another (crossing swords), thereby further impeding access to the surgical field (see Troubleshooting, pp. 90-91). Likewise, if the secondary sheaths are too near the initial laparoscopic sheath, the secondary sheath may ride over the primary sheath, again inhibiting access to the surgical field (e.g., "rollover").

In general, accessory trocars should be inserted at 90-degree angles to each other, forming an equilateral triangle or diamond array around the operative site (depending upon whether three or four trocars are used).

To align the secondary trocars better, it is helpful to use a marking pen to map out the proposed sites of introduction of the secondary trocars after insufflating the abdomen. The surgeon can then be certain that each point of entry is in a proper position to maximally aid the surgical procedure.

To avoid injury to any superficial abdominal wall vessels, the room lights are turned off and the proposed trocar sites are transilluminated with the laparoscope from inside the abdomen. The tip of the laparoscope is moved upward until it directly underlies the abdominal wall at the proposed trocar site (Fig. 7-1, A and B). At this point, it is helpful to change the light source from the video to manual setting to maximize the transmitted light, thereby providing effective transillumination. Larger superficial vessels can often be seen coursing just beneath the skin of the abdominal wall; the stab incision in the skin can thereby be made so as to avoid these vessels. When placing trocars in the lower

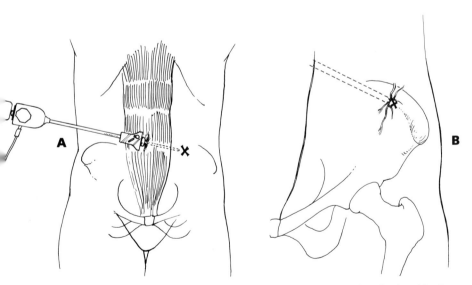

Fig. 7-1 A, Tip of the laparoscope is tilted upward until the tip lies flush with the anterior abdominal wall. Turn the setting on the light source from automatic to manual; adjust the brightness setting for maximal intensity. **B,** Skin incision for the trocar is made lateral to the transilluminated vessels of the abdominal wall.

abdominal quadrants, care must be taken to avoid injuring deeper abdominal wall vessels, specifically the inferior epigastric vessels. The location of the inferior epigastric vessels is identifiable as a short, band-like protrusion of the anterior peritoneum into the abdominal cavity; this area lies just lateral to the medial umbilical ligament and caudal and medial to the internal inguinal ring. Secondary trocars are purposely positioned either medial or lateral to the inferior epigastric vessels.

TROCAR INSERTION

The skin is incised transversely, just enough to accommodate the size of the trocar. A clamp can be used again to spread the incision cephalocaudally, thereby "rounding" out the incision so it will more easily accommodate the trocar. The incision for these ports, especially for the smaller 5 mm trocars, should be just through the skin; no attempt is made to nick the fascia. For this purpose a No. 12 (i.e., hook) blade is most helpful, because it is excellent for making and elongating the incision to the precise diameter of the trocar.

The trocar is held so that the middle or index finger of the dominant hand extends down the sheath of the trocar to act as a brake (see Chapter 5). If the trocar has a sidearm stopcock, it is turned to the *off* position.

All trocars should be introduced in a direct line with the planned surgical field so that after introduction, even when the sheath is not being held, the sheath will naturally point toward the surgical site. If this is not done, the sheath may end up pointing away from the surgical site. The surgeon will then have to place significant pressure on the sheath each time an instrument is passed in order to orient the instrument toward the surgical site. This is particularly bothersome in obese patients. Also, the additional force needed to redirect the sheath deprives the surgeon or surgical assistant of the deft touch and feel necessary to palpate tissues through the laparoscopic instruments (Fig. 7-2, *A* and *B*). In Fig. 7-2, *A*, a gallbladder procedure is planned. All of the ports are properly aligned. Each port is pointed toward the site of surgery. Similarly, all sheaths are placed so as to "surround" the surgical site as much as possible. In Fig. 7-2, *B*, the ports have been placed in a haphazard fashion, thereby making it more difficult for the surgeon to direct instruments to the surgical site.

Also, when a sheath is improperly inserted, the increased pressure necessary to redirect the sheath further tears the peritoneum, thereby resulting in a larger peritoneotomy, with attendant loss of the peritoneal seal against the sheath (Fig. 7-3, *A* and *B*). This results in continuous leakage of CO_2 from the abdominal cavity. Accordingly, a little forethought can preclude hours of difficulty.

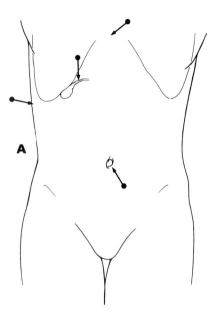

A

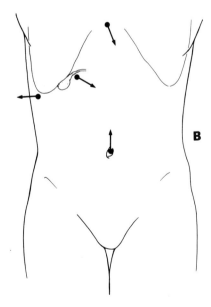

B

Fig. 7-2 **A,** For a gallbladder procedure, all trocars should be directed toward the surgical site. **B,** Random trocar direction results in difficulty delivering the instrumentation to the surgical site.

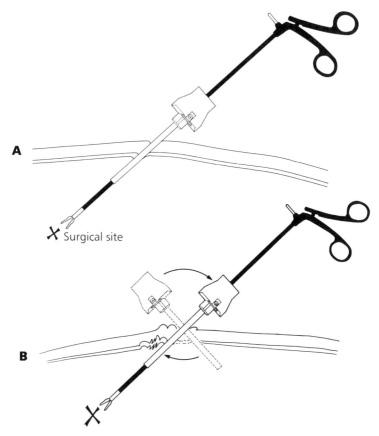

A

X Surgical site

B

X

Fig. 7-3 A, Proper trocar direction should be toward the operative site. **B,** If this is not done, the peritoneum will be torn, as the surgeon must force the trocar into a proper direction.

Under continuous laparoscopic monitoring, the secondary trocar is introduced into the skin with a slow, twisting action. The tip of the obturator is seen as it enters the peritoneal cavity. Further introduction of the obturator continues until the sheath completely enters the peritoneal cavity. During this part of the procedure, the surgeon can clearly see any underlying viscera on the television screen. If the sharp tip of the obturator is coming too close to the underlying bowel (Fig. 7-4, *A*), then the perpendicular angle of entry can be made more acute, either away from or toward the laparoscope (Fig. 7-4, *B* and *C*), thereby directing the sheath as it traverses the peritoneum, away from the bowel.

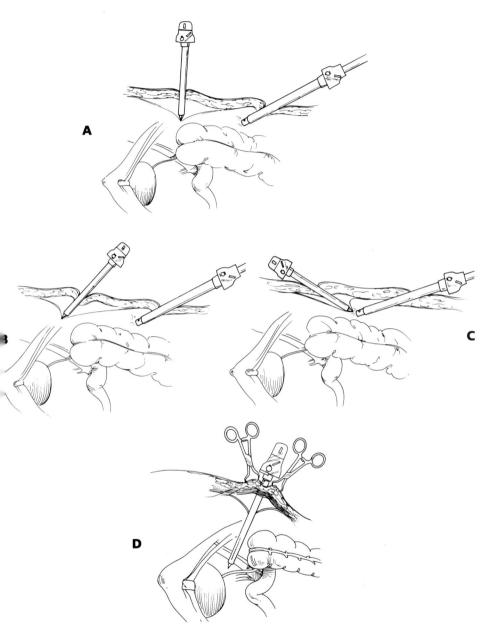

Fig. 7-4 A, Trocar coming too close to underlying viscera. **B,** Trocar directed away from laparoscope and more parallel to the abdominal wall. **C,** Towel clips applied to the skin to help lift the abdominal wall away from the underlying viscera. Trocar is successfully and safely inserted. **D,** Alternatively, the trocar is pointed directly at the 0-degree laparoscope; the trocar is advanced well above the viscera as the laparoscope is retracted until the trocar enters the abdominal cavity.

Also, the abdominal wall can be elevated manually or with towel clips (Fig. 7-4, *D*). When the obturator is removed, the fascia, which was traversed perpendicularly, will maintain the sheath in the original perpendicular position—thereby directing the sheath toward the surgical site.

SHEATH RETENTION

To prevent the laparoscopic sheaths (i.e., ports) from slipping out of the abdominal wall during the procedure an integral or detachable outer retentive groove can be helpful. The integral retentive sheath is introduced deeply into the abdomen. In contrast, the detachable retentive sleeve is introduced just until it appears in the abdominal cavity. With the detachable type of collar, the collar is advanced over the sheath with a twisting motion. Once the collar extends 2 cm into the abdomen, the sheath is retracted until it protrudes only 1 to 2 cm beyond the intraperitoneal end of the collar. The tightening bolt on the retentive collar is then secured, thereby fixing the collar to the sheath; now the sheath can be neither inadvertently advanced nor retracted.

NB: A *plastic* retentive sleeve should not be used in combination with a *metal* sheath; this is a potentially dangerous combination. The plastic retentive sleeve will insulate the metal sheath as it passes through the abdominal wall and act as a capacitor; any electrical current that inadvertently comes into contact with the metal sheath may spark to adjacent organs or bowel (Fig. 7-5, *A* and *B*). Normally, when the bare metal portion of the sheath is in direct contact with the abdominal wall, a "shorting out" of any transmitted electrical current occurs harmlessly over the broad surface of the abdominal wall where it is in contact with the metal sheath.

If a retentive sleeve or collar-type trocar is not available, another way to secure the secondary sheath is to tie the sidearm of the sheath to the abdominal skin with an 0-silk suture (Fig. 7-6). The sheath is retracted until only 2 cm of it protrudes into the abdominal cavity. The curved needle is passed through the skin immediately adjacent to the trocar. The suture is wrapped several times around the sidearm of the sheath and tied. Although the sheath can still be advanced deeper into the abdomen, it cannot be inadvertently pulled out of the peritoneal cavity.

PRIMARY TROCAR SITE INSPECTION

As soon as the initial secondary trocar is placed, a 10 mm or 5 mm endoscope is passed through the secondary sheath. *The entry site of the ≥10 mm initial trocar into the abdominal cavity is inspected to be certain that it has not traversed the omentum or a loop of bowel. If this has occurred,*

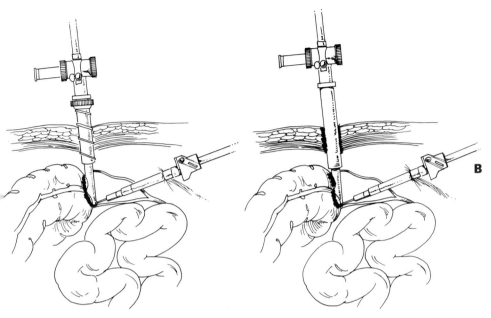

Fig. 7-5 **A,** Plastic retentive sleeve on a metal sheath acts as insulator and electrical energy is transferred to the bowel, thereby causing injury. **B,** Bare metal sheath allows electrical energy to dissipate along the abdominal wall, thereby decreasing conductance and subsequent injury to any viscera in contact with the laparoscopic metal sheath.

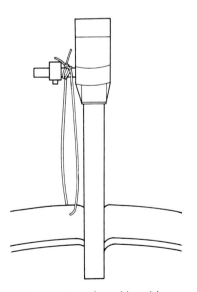

Fig. 7-6 Trocar secured to skin with a suture.

appropriate reparative maneuvers must be instituted (see Trouble-shooting, p. 98). At this time the sheath of the initial trocar can be repositioned so that it also protrudes only 2 cm into the abdominal cavity; a retentive sleeve or suture can now be used to fix the position of the initial sheath. Then the 10 mm laparoscope can be returned to the primary ≥10 mm sheath, and additional secondary trocars are placed again under direct endoscopic monitoring.

TROUBLESHOOTING: SECONDARY TROCAR PLACEMENT

Problem: Properitoneal fat is too thick and the peritoneum too mobile; the point of the trocar cannot be seen to enter the abdomen.
Solution:
- Via one or two of the other previously placed secondary sheaths, an instrument can be passed to help exert upward pressure on the abdominal wall at the point of planned trocar entry, thereby facilitating entry into the peritoneal cavity (abdominal lift maneuver).
- Use towel clips to stabilize and slightly elevate the trocar skin incision site.
- Direct the trocar more perpendicular to the skin.
- Slightly rotate the trocar through a 90-degree arc as it is passed through the tissues of the abdominal wall; do not vigorously twist it back and forth, because this may stretch the peritoneum, thereby making it even more lax and thus harder to puncture.
- Via another secondary port, incise the peritoneum where it is being pushed by the trocar.

Problem: *Crossing swords*. The intra-abdominal portions of two sheaths are too close to each other and cross one another; thus one sheath blocks mobility of the other sheath (Fig. 7-7, *A*).
Solution: The surgical cutting or dissecting instrument is best passed through a sheath that passes between two other trocar sites. In this way traction and countertraction can be placed on the tissue; the scissors can then be used to cut the tissue in between the two opposing graspers. If this is not done, tissue held by the two trocars may not be accessible to the cutting instrument. Likewise, if the tissue is not held taut, it will be more difficult to incise (Fig. 7-7, *B*). The graspers on the tissues should be used to pull the tissue in opposite directions while aligning the tissue as the scissors approach the tissue as perpendicularly as possible. If there is still difficulty in using the

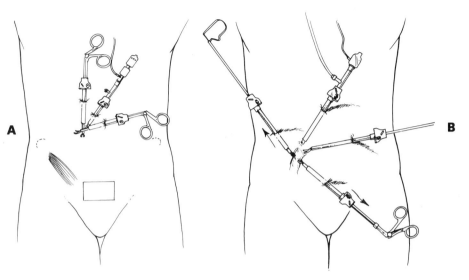

Fig. 7-7 A, Crossing swords. **B,** Proper instrument placement to achieve traction and countertraction before incising tissue: "traction/countertraction—cut in the middle."

trocars despite these maneuvers, consideration should be given to placing an additional 5 mm trocar distant from the two trocars that are striking one another. Both principles are demonstrated in Fig. 7-7, B.

Problem: *Striking handles* (Fig. 7-8, A). If this situation occurs, the secondary sheaths have been placed too close to each other and are positioned too deep within the abdomen. As such, the extra-abdominal portion of the sheaths will strike each other when instruments are passed.

Prevention: Before placing secondary trocars, mark the skin where they are to be placed. This will allow the surgeon to be certain of placing the trocars well away from each other. Plan your port placement; think geometrically: three ports = equilateral triangle, four ports = square, or five ports = pentagon.

Solution: Pull each sheath as far out of the abdomen as possible to allow a greater distance (i.e., wider arc) between the flap valve introduction portion of the two neighboring sheaths (Fig. 7-8, B).

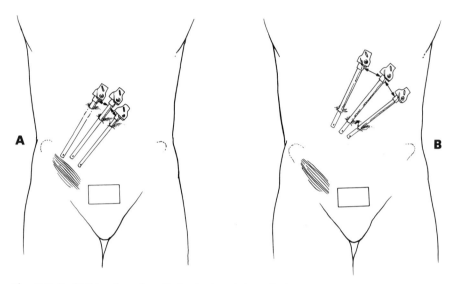

Fig. 7-8 **A,** Striking handles. **B,** Each sheath is pulled as far out of the abdomen as possible, thereby increasing the distance between the access port of each trocar.

Problem: *Rollover.* The laparoscope-containing primary sheath and one of the instrument-bearing secondary sheaths are directed toward one another rather than running parallel to the surgical field. Initially the vessel grasped is clearly seen (Fig. 7-9, *A* and *B*). However, as the 0-degree laparoscope is advanced deeper into the abdomen, it strikes the secondary sheath above the monitored surgical site (Fig. 7-9, *C*). The surgeon may notice the problem because either there is a physical resistance to advancing the laparoscope to the surgical field or the instrument seems to "roll over" an unseen obstacle (i.e., the 0-degree laparoscope). The view of the grasping forceps is thereby lost (Fig. 7-9, *D*).

Solution: The 0-degree laparoscope should be directed so it runs more parallel to the instrument-bearing sheath (Fig. 7-9, *E*); this will move the surgical site into one corner of the monitor (Fig. 7-9, *F*) but will decrease the rollover problem. Alternatively, a sheath further removed from the laparoscope can be selected for instrument passage or a new secondary trocar may be introduced.

■ Change to a 30-degree laparoscope. The rollover problem can be eliminated by rotating the *endoscope* (not the camera), 90 degrees

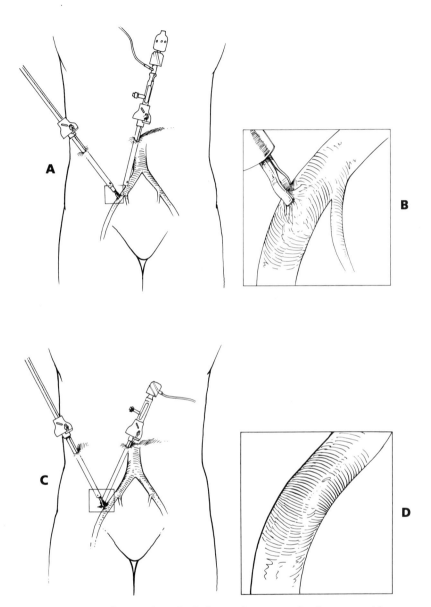

Fig. 7-9 A, Overview of procedure. **B,** 0-degree laparoscopic picture on video monitor of the vessel grasped, albeit at a distance. **C,** As the 0-degree laparoscope is moved closer to the site, the grasper is pushed over the shaft of the laparoscope (i.e., rollover). **D,** Grasper has rolled over the shaft of the 0-degree laparoscope and is no longer in view on the monitor.   *Continued.*

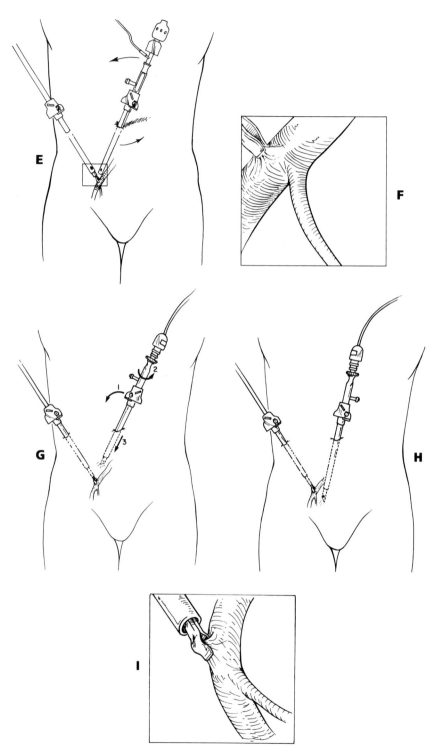

Fig. 7-9, cont'd E-I, For legend see opposite page.

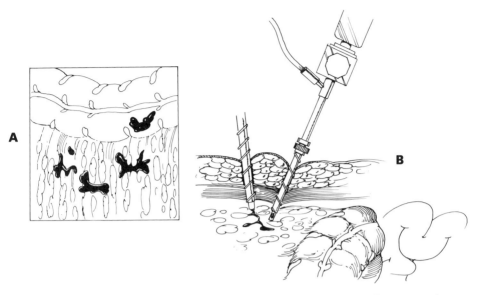

Fig. 7-10 A, Blood on omentum and bowel. **B,** Bleeding from secondary trocar site.

to the right or left, thereby providing a side view of the surgical field; simultaneously, the camera person can move the extra-abdominal camera end of the laparoscope toward the dominant instrument-bearing hand of the surgeon. The intra-abdominal tip of the laparoscope is moved away from the tip of the instrument it was striking, thereby eliminating the rollover problem.

Problem: Continuous stream of blood dripping from one of the trocars. Blood is seen on the bowel; examination of the secondary trocar site shows blood dripping from the secondary sheath (Fig. 7-10, *A* and *B*).

Solution: This problem usually is seen when one of the secondary trocars injures an inferior epigastric vessel. Identification of the ridge in the

---

Fig. 7-9, cont'd E, The 0-degree laparoscope is shifted so it lies more parallel to the grasper. **F,** This stops the rollover, but the area to be grasped is now viewed only in one corner of the monitor (i.e., off-center). **G** and **H,** With a 25-degree lens, the laparoscope can be moved closer to the secondary port *(1)* and advanced deeper into the abdomen *(3)* while the endoscope is rotated *(2)* 90 degrees. This provides a side view of the area of interest and eliminates the rollover problem. **I,** Side view of area of interest provided by the 25-degree lens.

anterior abdominal wall created by these vessels and avoidance of this area during direct, endoscopically monitored trocar placement are the best ways to prevent this annoying problem. To determine the point at which the vessel was injured, the trocar can be canti-levered into each of four quadrants (i.e., medial, lateral, cephalad, caudad) until the flow of blood is noted to cease (Fig. 7-11, *A* and *B*). A suture is then placed such that it traverses the entire border of the designated quadrant (Fig. 7-11, *C* and *D*).

A large curved No. 1 absorbable suture on an XXLH needle is used. The needle enters the abdomen on one side of the trocar and exits on the other side, thereby encircling the full thickness of the abdominal wall. The passage of the suture is monitored endoscop-ically.

In an obese person, a straight Keith needle may be substituted for the curved needle (Fig. 7-11, *C* and *D*). Laparoscopic needle holders are used to pull the needle into the abdomen on one side of the trocar; the needle is then transferred to a second laparoscopic needle holder and rotated until the tip is pointing at the undersurface of the abdominal wall. The needle is then pushed from inside the abdominal wall on the opposite side of the trocar until the needle's tip exits the skin. The needle is grasped and pulled out of the skin. The suture, which now encircles the full thickness of the abdominal wall, is tied over a gauze bolster (Fig. 7-11, *E*).

Problem: Tip of the obturator has pierced the peritoneum, but it lies dangerously close to the underlying viscera.
Solution:
- Towel clips are placed on either side of the skin site and used to lift up the skin to increase the distance between the tip of the obturator and underlying viscera.
- Increase pneumoperitoneum to 25 mm Hg.
- As a last resort, the obturator can be angled away from the un-derlying viscera so that it lies more *parallel* to the anterior abdominal wall. The trocar is then inserted deeper until it is completely within the abdominal cavity. Although this maneuver will preclude vis-ceral injury, it may result in larger peritoneotomy as the sheath is subsequently maneuvered in the abdomen (see Fig. 7-4, *A-C*). Al-ternatively, the trocar can be directed at the tip of the laparoscope; as the laparoscope is backed away the trocar is advanced until it is in the peritoneal cavity (i.e., "stick-the-scope" maneuver).

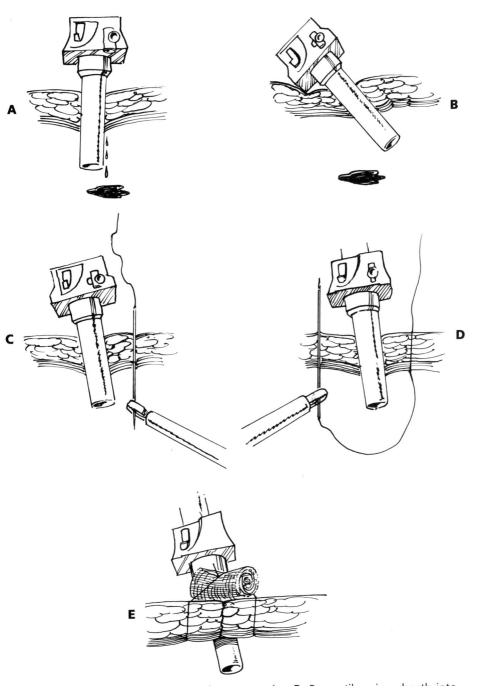

Fig. 7-11 A, Bleeding from secondary trocar site. **B,** By cantilevering sheath into each quadrant, a position of the sheath is found that causes the bleeding to stop. **C,** A straight needle is passed into the abdomen at the inferior border of this quadrant. **D,** The needle is reversed inside the abdomen and passed inside out through the abdominal wall at the superior border of the quadrant. **E,** The suture is tied securely over a gauze bolster, thereby stopping the bleeding.

Problem: Trocar injury. Bowel, two-wall through-and-through puncture (Fig. 7-12).

Solution: If this occurs at the time of placement of the primary ≥10 mm trocar, the injury may not be recognized until the end of the case, unless the surgeon, *as recommended,* routinely scans the initial port site as soon as a secondary trocar is placed. When this problem is recognized, there are four possible courses of action, depending on the surgeon's experience:

- Formal open laparotomy and bowel repair/resection
- Laparoscopic suture repair of bowel injury
- Laparoscopic resection of injured bowel and reanastomosis using laparoscopic GIA staplers
- Minilaparotomy, just large enough to deliver injured bowel segment for external repair or resection and reanastomosis

All of these options will fare better if the patient has had a complete antibiotic and mechanical bowel preparation before the procedure. If no bowel preparation was done, the abdomen should be irrigated with 4 to 10 L of saline with or without an added antibiotic agent, depending on the surgeon's preference. Irrigation is continued until no particulate matter is seen in the aspirated returns.

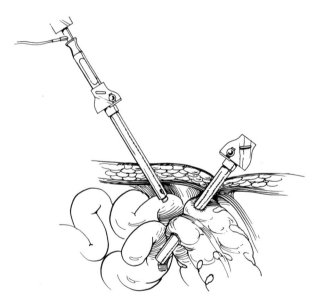

Fig. 7-12 Through-and-through bowel injury caused by initial trocar is recognized when the laparoscope is routinely moved to a secondary port to inspect the initial trocar site.

Problem: The tip of the obturator is seen entering the abdominal cavity, but the safety shield is not springing into the abdominal cavity (Fig. 7-13, *A*).

Prevention: When the trocar is first introduced, always be certain that the entire point of the obturator and the end of the safety shield clear the skin incision (Fig. 7-13, *B*).

Solution: The entire safety shield may not have traversed the skin. Thus the skin is holding the safety shield back and precluding its forward movement over the tip of the trocar. The skin incision may need to be extended.

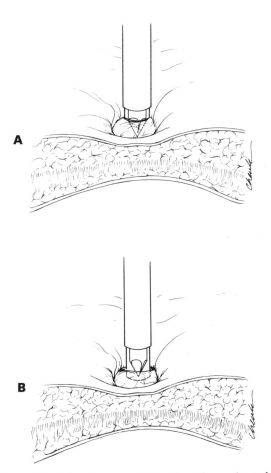

Fig. 7-13 A, The skin incision is too small to allow the entire safety shield to enter the skin; hence the trocar cannot be advanced. **B,** The entire safety shield has circumferentially entered the skin incision; the trocar can now be properly advanced.

Problem: Gas leak at trocar site (Fig. 7-14).
Solution:

- Purse-string suture around skin site (No. 2 nonabsorbable suture).
- Wrap petrolatum gauze around trocar at the skin site and then fix it with a suture to the trocar sheath.
- Turn inflow rate of CO_2 up to the maximal setting.
- Replace the trocar with a larger trocar (Fig. 7-15, *A-H*). Pass an appropriate-sized Amplatz fascial dilator through the trocar sheath and into the abdominal cavity *(A)*. Pass an 8 Fr Amplatz catheter through the Amplatz dilator *(B)* and pass a 0.035-inch Amplatz superstiff guidewire through the 8 Fr Amplatz catheter *(C)*. Remove the old trocar sheath *(D)*. Remove the obturator from the new, larger trocar. Proceed to use sequential Amplatz dilators to dilate the tract until the new, larger trocar sheath fits snugly over the last Amplatz dilator *(E-F)*. (A 5 mm trocar sheath = 16 Fr dilator; a 10 mm trocar sheath = 30 Fr dilator.) Slide the larger trocar sheath over the appropriate Amplatz dilator until the sheath is seen to enter the abdominal cavity *(G)*. Sew the sheath in place with a No. 2 nonabsorbable skin suture. Now remove the Amplatz dilator, 8 Fr Amplatz catheter, and guidewire *(H)*. Properly position the sheath and sew it in place.

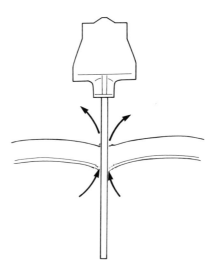

Fig. 7-14 Gas leak around trocar.

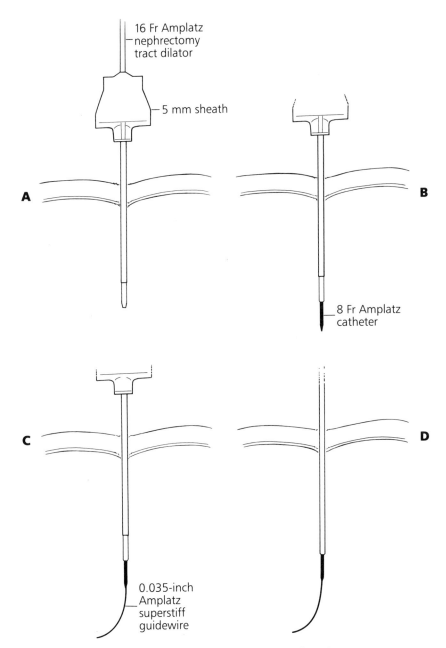

Fig. 7-15 A-H, Exchanging a small (i.e., 5 mm) trocar for a larger trocar to stop a peritrocar gas leak. *Continued.*

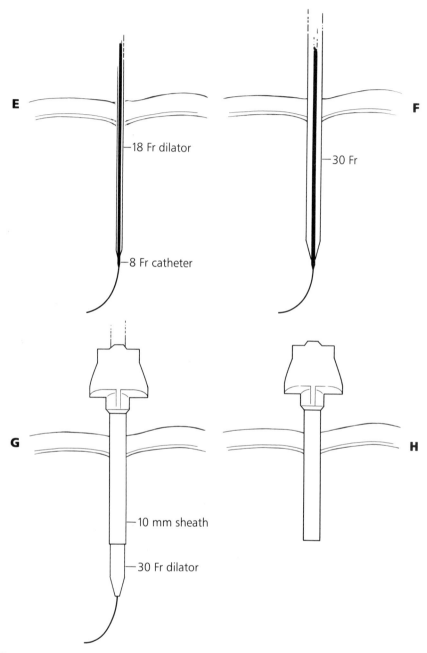

Fig. 7-15, cont'd Exchanging a small (i.e., 5 mm) trocar for a larger trocar to stop a peritrocar gas leak.

Problem: The ≥10 mm trocar seems too short to enter the abdominal cavity. This usually occurs in the lower midline of the abdomen if there is a particularly prominent urachus.

Solution:

- Place a 5 mm port in either the right or left lower quadrant, just lateral to the rectus muscle. Use a 5 mm laparoscope to examine the intra-abdominal contents. The most likely scenario is that the ≥10 mm port has been introduced at too acute an angle to the skin, thereby causing it to traverse a long expanse of properitoneal fat. The sheath is withdrawn, and the trocar is rearmed and passed perpendicular to the skin site. Under endoscopic monitoring the ≥10 mm trocar is advanced into the peritoneal cavity.
- Use any other ports in the abdomen to pass an instrument and push the peritoneal and properitoneal fat anteriorly, thereby providing counterpressure to the advancing trocar.

Problem: Trocar injury: omentum, through-and-through.

Recognition: The hallmark of this injury is blood dripping down the sheath and landing either on the surgical field or on the shaft and lens of the laparoscope. In the latter circumstance, the view through the laparoscope is continually being blurred shortly after placement of the laparoscope through the sheath. The injury is recognized during inspection of the primary trocar site via one of the secondary ports.

Solution: The laparoscope is withdrawn, cleansed, and reintroduced. The abdominal contents are inspected. If an omental injury is noted, a secondary port is placed and the site of injury is electrocoagulated. If no injury is noted, yet the lens is again clouded by blood, the laparoscope is again removed, cleansed, and a secondary trocar is introduced. A laparoscope is passed into the secondary sheath to examine the entry point of the primary ≥10 mm sheath into the abdomen. The problem is corrected by slowly pulling the ≥10 mm sheath out of the omentum and electrocoagulating any bleeding omental vessels.

CHAPTER 8

Laparoscopic Equipment

David S. Goldstein, Paramjit S. Chandhoke,
Louis R. Kavoussi, and Randall R. Odem

The success of laparoscopic surgery is highly reliant on equipment. This greater dependence on technology results from several factors. First, laparoscopic surgery does not afford the surgeon the three-dimensional view obtained during open exploration. Instead, the view through the laparoscope results in markedly diminished depth perception. Furthermore, the wide visual field normally available to assess anatomic relationships is not present. In addition, instrument movement is limited by fixation at the trocar entry site. Finally, the tactile sensation normally available to the surgeon through the hand-held instrument is blunted because of the passage of the instrument through the trocar and its valve.

Surgeons are still exploring the boundaries of this operative technique, and novel instrumentation is constantly being developed to parallel the newly conceived applications. Accordingly, to perform laparoscopic surgery safely and effectively, one must be completely familiar with each piece of this specialized equipment. The purpose of this chapter is to familiarize the surgeon with the basic instrumentation needed and available to perform laparoscopy.

Laparoscopic equipment can be subdivided into seven categories: insufflation system, trocars, optical system, documentation system, auxiliary instruments, irrigation/aspiration system, and other operative instrumentation (Appendices A-1 through A-7). A variety of laparoscopic equipment is available in each of these categories from many manufacturers. A complete list of manufacturers with their addresses and phone numbers is provided in Appendix A-8.

EQUIPMENT CARE

Proper handling and maintenance of all laparoscopic equipment will prove invaluable in terms of equipment reliability, availability, and costs. All of the large items should be stored in a portable cart. When equipment is moved from one operating room to another, the person pushing the cart should be extremely careful to avoid collisions with doors, bumps from elevators, and so on. In addition, the cart should be locked when not in use, limiting access to both the buttons on the front of the equipment and the cord connections on the back.

It is imperative that those responsible for cleaning and sterilizing understand how the instruments are taken apart, as well as how to correctly reassemble them. This understanding avoids a lot of equipment breakage; when the assembly is not understood, one frequently uses a clamp to force, loosen, or tighten. This usually breaks or strips the equipment and also frequently damages the clamp. Lenses and light cables should be handled carefully to avoid breakage and scratches. Reusable needles and trocars should be kept sharp. A system in which the trocars are sent for sharpening on a rotating basis will assure an adequate supply of sharp instruments. While the instruments are being cleaned, they should be inspected for mechanical defects, problems with insulation, or any other flaws. When problems are identified, the equipment should be sent for repair or, if necessary, should be replaced. If there is not an immediate replacement available, surgeons must be made aware of the deficiency before starting an operation so that there are no unexpected intraoperative equipment shortages.

Each section in this chapter has specific guidelines concerning relevant equipment care and maintenance. Following these guidelines will add significantly to the life expectancy of the equipment and greatly reduce operating room costs.

INSUFFLATION SYSTEM

The insufflation system allows the surgeon to obtain and maintain a pneumoperitoneum. The major components are the insufflant, the insufflator, and the insufflation needle.

Insufflant

Over the decades various gases have been used for laparoscopy. The first was room air. Because air is insoluble in blood, only relatively small amounts of gas can safely enter the bloodstream. As such, the use of filtered room air as an insufflant can result in an air embolus; thus air is no longer recommended as an insufflant. The use of oxygen has been avoided because of the risk of explosion in the presence of electrosurgical instrumentation. Other gases such as xenon, argon, and krypton have very desirable qualities for a laparoscopic insufflant (i.e., highly soluble in blood, inert, nonflammable), but these gases are not routinely used because of their cost.

Currently the two gases used most often for laparoscopic insufflation are carbon dioxide (CO_2) and nitrous oxide (N_2O). Of these two, CO_2 is preferred for all but short diagnostic procedures. When absorbed, CO_2 rapidly dissolves in blood, thereby decreasing the risk of gas embolism. Furthermore, CO_2 does not support combustion, so electrosurgical instruments can be used safely in its presence.

The main drawbacks of CO_2 are that it is a peritoneal irritant and when it is absorbed significant acidosis can result. CO_2 is converted to carbonic acid both on the peritoneal surface and in the bloodstream. The former situation may cause diaphragmatic irritation and postoperative pain; the latter situation results in metabolic acidosis.

Because of these shortcomings some laparoscopists prefer to use N_2O as the insufflant, especially for short procedures. N_2O is not a peritoneal irritant and when absorbed does not result in metabolic abnormalities. However, *it is less soluble in blood than CO_2* and theoretically presents a higher risk for gas embolism. Moreover, there is a small but real risk of problems if N_2O is used in the presence of electrosurgical instruments, since it can support combustion.

Insufflator

The insufflator consists of a sophisticated valve mechanism that gates the flow of the pressurized gas from the tank into the patient's abdomen. Currently several companies produce electronically controlled insufflators. All insufflators have standard functions that can be adjusted and monitored (Fig. 8-1). The gauges indicate rate of flow (given in

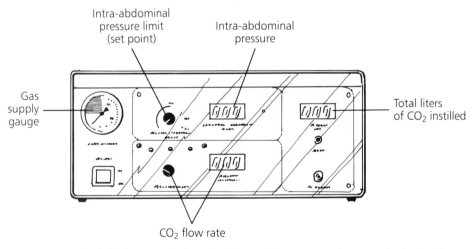

Fig. 8-1 Typical display panel of an insufflator. The gas supply gauge indicates the amount of CO_2 in the gas tank. Other displays indicate the pressure in the peritoneal cavity, the rate of gas inflow, the intra-abdominal pressure limit, and the total amount of gas used during the procedure.

liters per minute), intra-abdominal pressure (millimeters of mercury), and total liters of gas insufflated. A separate indicator measures the line pressure of the gas tank. Tank pressures >500 psi register in the green, indicating that an adequate amount of gas is present in the tank to perform laparoscopy. Gas is transported from the insufflator to the patient by flexible, inert sterile tubing.

The flow control varies the rate of CO_2 delivery into the patient's abdomen. Some units have only three settings: low (1 L/min), medium, or high (6 to 10 L/min) flow rates; others can be adjusted from 1 to 15 L/min in increments of 0.1 L/min. During initiation of the pneumoperitoneum, low flow rates (1 L/min) are used. If insufflation is proceeding properly, then after 1 L of CO_2 has entered the abdomen, the flow can be increased to $\geq$6 L/min.

The intra-abdominal pressure (mm Hg) is monitored by the insufflator and registered on an analog or digital gauge. The surgeon should be constantly aware of the intra-abdominal pressure throughout the procedure; accordingly, the insufflator should be placed just beneath the surgeon's monitor so it is always clearly visible. At high intra-abdominal pressures (>25 mm Hg) the patient is at increased risk of gas absorption, decreased venous return from the inferior vena cava, impaired ventilation as a result of pressure on the diaphragm, and the development of systemic acidosis. All modern-day insufflators can be set so that the flow of gas ceases when a predetermined intra-abdominal pressure is achieved. For most adult laparoscopic procedures, the set point is 15 mm Hg. Without this "cut-off" feature, the laparoscopic procedure becomes much more dangerous, since the surgeon must be ever vigilant of any changes in the intra-abdominal pressure.

Insufflation needle

The most common needle used for insufflation of the peritoneal cavity is the 14-gauge (6 Fr or 2 mm diameter) Veress needle (Fig. 8-2). The needle is used to penetrate the peritoneal cavity and deliver the gas into the abdomen. Standard needle lengths are 12 and 15 cm.

The Veress needle consists of a protruding, hollow, inner blunt tip and a sharp, recessed, outer beveled sheath. The inner blunt tip is spring-loaded so that it will retract when it meets resistance, thus exposing the sharp outer beveled sheath (e.g., when pushing on the abdominal wall fascia). As the needle is advanced, the sharp sheath penetrates the fascia and then punctures the peritoneum; once this

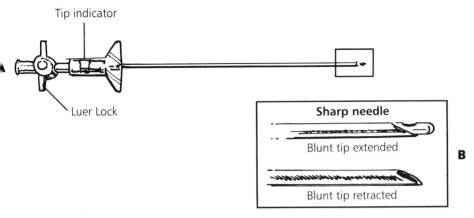

Fig. 8-2 A, Veress needle. **B,** Inset, the tip has an inner blunt core that retracts when encountering resistance from tissue but pops forward once the needle is in the peritoneal cavity (i.e., no resistance). The hub of this disposable plastic needle contains a red marker that shows the position of the blunt tip of the inner core relative to the needle tip.

resistance is overcome (i.e., by entering the peritoneal cavity), the spring-loaded, retracted, inner blunt tip moves forward, thereby projecting beyond the sharp tip of needle and thus protecting non-tethered underlying abdominal structures from inadvertent injury. Some Veress needles contain a red marker on the handle of the needle that indicates whether the inner blunt core of the tip is extended or retracted.

The hub of the needle contains a Luer Lock connector for attachment to the insufflation tubing. Most needles also have a one-way stopcock built into the Luer Lock connector so that the flow of gas into the abdomen can be turned off if desired.

Both disposable and reusable Veress-type insufflating needles are available. The reusable needles tend to be made of metal and become dull with repeated use. Periodic sharpening is essential. The reusable needles can be disassembled for cleaning and sharpening; therefore it is important to be certain that all components of a reusable needle are tightened before use.

In contrast, the disposable needles are reliably sharp, constructed largely of plastic, and tend to be *lighter* than their reusable metal counterparts. These disposable needles provide the surgeon with a greater sense of "touch" as the needle traverses the various fatty, fascial, and peritoneal layers of the abdominal wall.

TROCARS

Trocars give the surgeon access to the peritoneal cavity. They are designed to serve two important functions. First, they are a means to maintain the pneumoperitoneum once the Veress needle is removed. All initially placed trocars and many secondary trocars have Luer Lock sidearm valves that can be attached to the insufflator tubing to allow continued gas flow into the peritoneum. Next, most trocars contain a valve mechanism or a series of seals built into the handle to prevent gas from escaping from the abdomen when the surgeon passes or removes an instrument, removes tissue from the abdomen, or withdraws the laparoscope.

Laparoscopic trocars consist of two components: a hollow outer sheath and a sharp inner obturator (Fig. 8-3, A). The pointed tip of the obturator may be conical (Fig. 8-3, B) or pyramidal (Fig. 8-3, C) in shape. The sharp obturator pierces the fascia and peritoneum, carrying with it the outer sheath. Once in the peritoneal cavity, the obturator is removed, leaving the sheath in place in the abdominal cavity.

Disposable and nondisposable trocars are available from a variety of manufacturers. The nondisposable trocars are made of metal and thus are heavier than their plastic disposable counterparts. They are also radiopaque, which is a disadvantage if intraoperative fluoroscopy or radiographs are needed. Also, the valve in the metal trocars is of a trumpet type and must be meticulously disassembled, cleaned, and reassembled before each procedure. Furthermore, the valve must be held or squeezed open while passing instruments into the abdomen; this is tiresome for the assistant and contributes to loss of CO_2 during the procedure. Finally, the tips of the nondisposable obturators tend to dull with use and need to be sharpened periodically.

In contrast, the disposable trocars are made of plastic and are thus lightweight. Another feature of the disposable trocars is the plastic safety shield that covers the sharp obturator. Similar in this respect to a Veress needle, the outer atraumatic shield of the obturator retracts as the assembled trocar is pushed against the abdominal wall, thereby exposing the sharp tip of the obturator (Fig. 8-4, A). As the obturator pierces the peritoneum and enters the gas-filled abdomen, the sudden loss of resistance allows the outer safety shield to spring forward and lock in place, covering the sharp tip of the obturator (Fig. 8-4, B) and

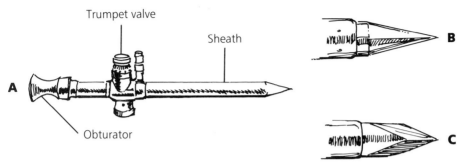

Fig. 8-3 A, Reusable trocar with trumpet valve. The tip of the obturator can be either conical, **B,** or pyramidal, **C.**

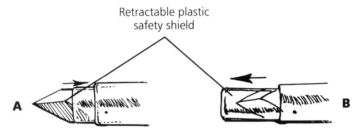

Fig. 8-4 Disposable trocar with a safety shield. The safety shield retracts, **A,** when resistance from tissue (such as fascia) is encountered; the spring-loaded shield moves forward and locks when the trocar enters the gas-filled peritoneal cavity, **B,** thereby covering the sharp tip of the obturator and precluding injury to the underlying viscera.

protecting the underlying abdominal organs from injury. The position (locked versus unlocked) of the safety shield at any given time is indicated by a spring-loaded red marker on the handle.

Most trocars have two valve mechanisms built into the handle. The first is an external stopcock with a Luer Lock fitting. This can be attached to the insufflation tubing to allow for maintenance of the pneumoperitoneum. The second valve mechanism lies in line with the lumen of the trocar and prevents loss of pneumoperitoneum when no instrument is in the trocar. In the disposable trocar, this is usually a flap valve that can be manually opened by a lever on the handle (Fig. 8-5, *A*). The closed (at rest) flap valve will readily open as pressure from the tip of an instrument is applied to it.

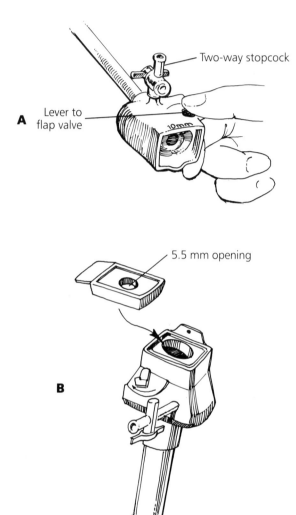

Fig. 8-5 A, Disposable trocar sheath with flap valve. When withdrawing sharp instruments such as hook electrodes or large pieces of tissue, the flap valve is opened using the lever on the handle to prevent damage to the valve mechanism or loss of the tissue specimen, respectively. **B,** Reducer.

Escape of gas around an instrument is prevented by a series of additional seals in the handle. When removing certain instruments (e.g., a hook electrode) or when removing tissue, it is necessary to hold the valve in its open position.

In some of the newer, less expensive trocars, there is no sidearm stopcock. These trocars can be used only as secondary working trocars for the passage of auxiliary instrumentation. The sheath valve is a penetrable plastic membrane that seals only when an instrument is passed through it. When no instrument is in the sheath, a finger must be placed over the end of the sheath to prevent loss of the pneumoperitoneum.

Standard trocars are available in diameters ranging from 3 to 15 mm; some newly developed trocars are as large as 30 mm. The 5 mm diameter trocars allow for passage of most working instruments, including electrosurgical probes, graspers, scissors, forceps, needle drivers, and smaller laparoscopes. The larger 10 to 12 mm ports are for placement of clip appliers, specialized staplers, standard size laparoscopes (10 mm), and tissue morcellators. These larger ports are also better suited for tissue removal from the abdominal cavities. The 30 mm ports are currently used to perform laparoscopically assisted bowel surgery.

The working length of the trocar is measured from the end of the trocar sheath to the hub on the sheath. Trocars come in working lengths ranging from 5 to 15 cm; the shorter trocars are used in children, and the longer ones are used in obese adults. The working length of a standard 5 mm diameter trocar is approximately 7 cm and that of a 10 mm diameter trocar is 11 cm.

Specially designed *reducers* are available to downsize the larger ≥10 mm trocars to permit use of smaller 5 mm instruments without allowing gas to escape from the abdomen. These reducers fit either on top of the trocar or are gasketed long tubes placed inside the sheath; each type of fitted reducer is specific to a particular type of trocar (Fig. 8-5, B).

A problem that frequently arises during laparoscopy is inadvertent removal of a trocar sleeve from the peritoneal cavity. Attempts to minimize the risk of dislodging a trocar have resulted in several design alterations in both nondisposable (i.e., reusable) and disposable trocars. Specifically, nondisposable trocars have been made with a roughened shaft to increase resistance between the tissues of the abdominal wall and the side of the trocar. In contrast, disposable trocars have been created with separate outer threaded sleeves that can be affixed to the sheath and can then be screwed into the abdominal wall to prevent the

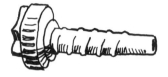

Fig. 8-6 A disposable outer plastic sheath can be backloaded and affixed to the sheath of a plastic trocar. The *threaded sleeves* are screwed into the abdominal wall to prevent inadvertent removal of the laparoscopic sheath during the procedure. Use of this plastic covering in conjunction with a metal sheath is not recommended (see Fig. 7-5, *A*).

sheath from being pulled out (Fig. 8-6). Although effective, this method makes it difficult to vary the depth of the trocar sheath within the peritoneal cavity during the procedure. Moreover, gas can track around the threads, resulting in subcutaneous emphysema. Other retention-type disposable trocars have a Malecot-type design in the tip so that on withdrawal of the obturator, the wings of the Malecot expand, thereby "locking" the sheath into the abdomen. An outer sliding ring can then be locked onto the sleeve of the trocar at the skin level to fix the sheath so it cannot be retracted or advanced inadvertently. By loosening the outer ring, the operator can adjust the amount of sheath protruding into the abdomen. Finally, other trocar sheaths have a balloon on the tip of the sheath. Once the sheath is inserted in the abdomen, the balloon can be expanded within the abdomen to secure the sheath in place.

A simpler alternative to secure the sheath is to use a No. 2 nonabsorbable suture to anchor the trocar sleeve to the abdominal wall. The trocar is pulled back under laparoscopic guidance so that its tip extends approximately 2 cm into the peritoneal cavity. Then the suture is passed through the abdominal skin; the two loose ends of the suture are wrapped twice about the insufflation valve and tied. This suture allows the trocar to be advanced deeper into the abdomen but precludes its inadvertent removal.

In certain patients (e.g., those with multiple prior abdominal surgeries or obese individuals), open trocar placement may be necessary. A specially designed open cannula (e.g., Hasson) works well in this situation (Fig. 8-7). The cannula consists of a blunt-tipped obturator and a conical outer adjustable sleeve on the sheath. For open placement,

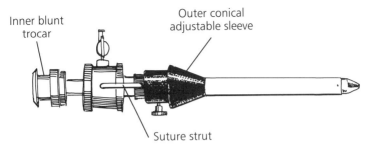

Fig. 8-7 Open (e.g., Hasson) cannula. This cannula is placed within the peritoneal cavity under *direct vision* after a peritoneal incision has been made. The trocar sheath is anchored in place with fascial sutures that are fixed to the sheath's struts.

a 2 cm incision is made in the abdominal wall down through fascia. Two stay sutures (0-absorbable) are placed, one in either side of the fascial incision. The peritoneum is then incised, and the underside of the abdominal wall is probed with a finger to be sure that neither bowel nor omentum is adherent. The obturator of the open cannula is then inserted into the peritoneotomy; the outer conical sleeve is moved forward and pushed tightly into the fascial opening and secured to the sheath by a set screw. The previously placed stay sutures are then put on traction and affixed to the struts on the sheath of the cannula or on the cone-shaped sleeve, thereby forming a tight seal between the fixed outer conical sleeve and the peritoneum. The blunt-tipped obturator is then removed. At the end of the procedure, the two fascial sutures can be tied to each other, thereby easily closing the fasciotomy.

OPTICAL SYSTEM

The optical system allows the surgeon to visualize the operative field within the abdominal cavity. This system consists of the laparoscope, camera/monitor, and light source.

Laparoscope

The laparoscope is the endoscope through which light and an image are transmitted from the peritoneal cavity directly through a camera and to the television monitor. The modern laparoscope consists of a rigid rod-lens imaging system (objective lens, rod-lens system, with or

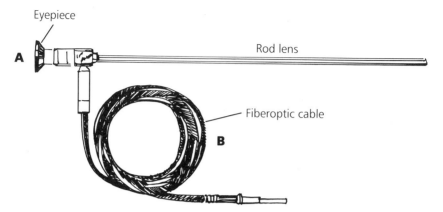

Fig. 8-8 Laparoscope. **A,** This consists of an objective lens, a rod-lens system, an eyepiece for image transmission, and internal fiberoptic bundles for light transmission. **B,** The light post of the endoscope is attached to a fiberoptic light cable.

without an eyepiece lens) and a fiberoptic light-conducting cable (Fig. 8-8).

The objective lens at the tip of the endoscope gathers the light that has been reflected by the tissue and focuses the inverted image on the end of the rod-lens system. The rod-lens system is a series of long glass lenses separated by short air spaces that transmits the image and reverses it at the eyepiece; the image is then magnified and transferred to the camera and then the television monitor.

The fiberoptic light cable within the laparoscope runs from the light post fitting to the tip of the laparoscope; the light cord fits into the light post on the laparoscope and transmits light from the light source. If the light coming from the tip of the endoscope appears dull, the light cord should be checked separately, and then with it connected to the laparoscope. Any interruption in the ring of light emanating from the tip of the light cable or from the tip of the endoscope is indicative of broken optical fibers within the light cord or endoscope, respectively.

Endoscopes are available in several diameters ranging from 2.7 to 12 mm. The most commonly used diameter for therapeutic laparoscopy is the 10 mm laparoscope. The larger laparoscopes are capable of transmitting a greater amount of light, and they provide a slightly wider field of view and supply a higher quality resolution than the smaller endoscopes.

The optical system most commonly used is a 0- or 5-degree lens; however, for certain applications endoscopes that provide an oblique view are available—that is, 30- and 45-degree angles. The 30- and 45-degree lenses are particularly helpful for viewing adhesions, the anterior abdominal wall, or for "looking over" a shelf of tissue. With the 30- and 45-degree endoscopes the field is as one would see it at open surgery when the light post is upright. As the light post and endoscope, but not the camera, are rotated, a sideview of the surgical site can be obtained. In contrast, rotating a 0-degree lens laparoscope (but *not* the camera) does not change the orientation at all.

Some laparoscopes are available with a built-in working channel. These "operating" laparoscopes provide optical information and also allow the surgeon to pass an instrument or laser beam directly into the field. Unfortunately, the working channel uses space ordinarily reserved for the optical system; thus the monitor image is inferior compared with a nonoperating endoscope of the same diameter. These laparoscopes are convenient for minor procedures in which a single trocar is adequate.

Camera/video system

The camera system is essential in performing effective diagnostic and therapeutic laparoscopy. It has completely replaced "direct" vision laparoscopy. The camera magnifies the endoscopic image, thereby allowing excellent visualization of very fine anatomic details. Moreover, the video monitor (i.e., television) provides an excellent view of the surgical field to all operating room personnel. This facilitates the surgery by permitting the assistants, scrub nurse, and anesthesiologist to stay abreast of the procedure. Also, the camera system can be attached to a documentation system to provide a visual record of the surgical pathology or to be used later to develop teaching aids for patients and medical personnel.

The camera system consists of the camera and a video monitor. The camera locks onto the eyepiece of the endoscope (Fig. 8-9). The camera receives the optical information from the endoscope and transmits it via a cable to the camera box; the image is then reconstructed and sent to the video monitor where the optical information is displayed (Fig. 8-10, *A* and *B*). When attaching the camera to the eyepiece, one must be certain that the endoscope and the camera eyepiece are clean and *free of moisture*, or "fogging" of the image will occur. In recently available camera systems, the camera is directly integrated into the optical system

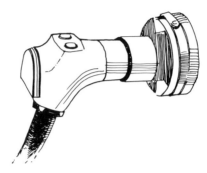

Fig. 8-9 Camera. The camera is attached to the eyepiece of the laparoscope.

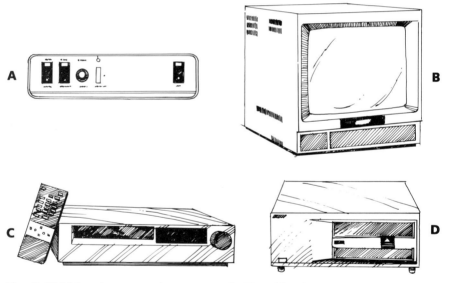

Fig. 8-10 Video documentation system. **A,** The video image is captured by the camera and camera box unit and is subsequently displayed, **B,** on a high-resolution video monitor. **C,** This in turn may be connected to a VCR for recording purposes. **D,** Selected images may be printed for documentation with a video printer.

of the endoscope; hence there is no eyepiece. This direct coupling of endoscope and camera is beneficial because it eliminates the lens/camera interface problem and improves the image quality as more light is transmitted directly to the surgical field.

The camera image should be oriented on the video monitor so that it is upright (i.e., identical to what would be seen if the surgery were being performed through an abdominal incision). The surgeon must know in which position the camera should be held to obtain an upright image during dissection. Each camera has an orientation mark that when placed at the 12 o'clock position allows the surgeon to orient the image properly (i.e., "true"). The camera should then be locked to the endoscope in this position to maintain the proper orientation throughout the procedure. This is true regardless of whether a 0-, 30-, or 45-degree lens is being used.

Most cameras can be gas sterilized. Liquid sterilization of the camera can also be done if so stated by the manufacturer of the camera; however, this is harder on the camera than gas sterilization and should be avoided when possible. Alternatively, there are protective sterile plastic sleeves available that can be used to cover the camera head and cable to help prevent contamination of the sterile field. In these cases, the camera is bathed with 100% ethanol just before it is placed in the plastic sleeve.

Before the laparoscope is placed into the abdominal cavity, it is important to make sure the camera is focused and that the color scheme on the monitor is accurate. To focus and white-balance the camera, the camera should be attached to an illuminated laparoscope that is pointed at a white object (e.g., gauze sponge). The camera can then be focused so that the strands of the gauze sponge are sharp and clear on the monitor. Next, there is usually a single button on the camera box that can be pressed to white-balance the camera image. Some cameras are now available with an automatic white-balance feature.

Distortion of the camera image may be caused by several problems. First, when a cold endoscope is placed into the peritoneal cavity, moisture precipitates on the end of the lens system. This produces a hazy image ("fog"). To prevent this condensation, the endoscope can be warmed (e.g., by bathing it in warm water) before insertion into the abdomen. Another helpful measure is to use a commercially available antifog agent on the lens tip of the endoscope. The antifog agents can be applied to the tip of the laparoscope to prevent moisture from precipitating on the lens system. Also, as previously noted, occasionally moisture may be present on the eyepiece lens or on the camera; this will also cause a hazy image. As such, both the eyepiece and the camera should be dried thoroughly before tightly coupling them together and covering them with a plastic camera wrap. This plastic wrapper is secured to the laparoscope with two wire twist ties, thus lessening the chances of moisture entering the lens/camera interface during the procedure.

Video monitors come from a variety of manufacturers and are available in several standard sizes. The larger (19-inch) monitors provide a larger picture but poorer image resolution than the smaller (13-inch) monitors. Standard video monitors have 525 lines of resolution. Newer models have resolution capabilities of 1125 lines; this results in a clearer image. However, to take advantage of improvements in monitor resolution, the monitor must be coupled to a camera capable of providing the appropriate input.

Occasionally problems with visualization may be caused by a damaged camera cable, malfunctioning camera box, or damaged television monitor. Each piece of imaging equipment should be checked thoroughly before initiating laparoscopy.

Light source

Laparoscopic light sources are of the high-intensity variety. These light sources use a xenon, mercury, or halogen vapor bulb and have an output of 250 to 300 watts. They provide bright, even illumination. Some light sources have a built-in second bulb; however, extra bulbs should always be available to avoid any problems.

The light output intensity is controlled at the source. Too much illumination may wash out the image. Proper light intensity affords better depth perception and image detail. Dome units are equipped with automatic light-level adjustment. These units automatically increase light intensity if the light reaching the camera is too low and likewise decrease the light intensity when the light coming to the camera is too bright. Some light sources also have built-in flash capability, which is helpful for taking still photographs.

Light is transported from the light source to the laparoscope by a fiberoptic cable. These cables are flexible and must be sterilized before use. The light cord is both laparoscope- and source-specific, and it is important that all connections fit properly and tightly. If the connection is loose, a significant loss in the light reaching the surgical field will occur.

Light cords must be handled with care. Rough handling can result in breakage of the delicate optical fibers within the light cord, thereby decreasing light transmission. The integrity of the light cord can be checked before the procedure by plugging it into the light source. Light should come evenly from the end of the light cord; any dark areas indicate broken fibers.

DOCUMENTATION SYSTEM

Documentation of a laparoscopic procedure may be accomplished in a global or select fashion with a videocassette recorder (VCR) as well as a video printer (Fig. 8-10, *C* and *D*). Standard VCR units are available that use either a ½-inch or a ¾-inch tape. Better resolution is achieved with a ¾-inch tape; however, this tape size is not compatible with most home video sets. Recently super VHS ½-inch units have become available that are equivalent in quality to the ¾-inch tape units; however, the tape must be played on a super VHS recorder to appreciate the improvement.

Video printers are available; these attachments will reproduce any image displayed on a monitor, whether transmitted directly by the laparoscope or by a prerecorded videotape. One, four, and nine separate pictures can be stored in the printer's memory and reproduced on the same or several hard copies. Video disk recorders are also available; these machines can record and store hundreds of images on an optical disk. By storing images the disk can be reviewed and the printer can be used to produce a hard copy of selected images only.

AUXILIARY INSTRUMENTATION

A wide assortment of instruments is available to facilitate all types of laparoscopic surgical procedures. These instruments are available in both disposable and nondisposable models (i.e., reusable). In general, laparoscopic instruments must be of a sufficient diameter to allow passage through a given trocar sleeve and of sufficient length to reach the surgical site. Most standard laparoscopic instruments are 5 or 10 mm in diameter and 35 cm in length. Instruments for suturing and for placing clips and staples are thoroughly discussed in Chapters 9 and 10, respectively.

Grasping instruments

Laparoscopic grasping instruments are available in diameters ranging from 3 to 12 mm. Many of these instruments are insulated so that they can be connected to electrosurgical units to coagulate tissue that has been grasped (Fig. 8-11).

Most instruments have a scissors-type handle. The handles contain rings through which the thumb and ring finger may be passed similar to holding a surgical scissors. By separating the handles, the jaws of the instrument are opened and by bringing the handles together, the jaws of the instrument are closed (Fig. 8-12).

The opening mechanism of most instruments is either single action (only one jaw moves when opened) or double action (both jaws move) (Fig. 8-13). The double-action mechanism is preferable for dissection.

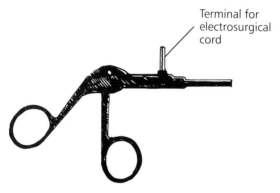

Terminal for electrosurgical cord

Fig. 8-11 Insulated instrument handle with a terminal for attachment of an electrosurgical cord.

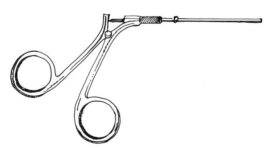

Fig. 8-12 Scissors-handle mechanism for opening and closing the jaws of an instrument.

Several mechanisms have been developed for locking the jaws in a closed position. Spring-loaded locking handles fit in the surgeon's palm and are opened by squeezing the handle (Fig. 8-14). This type of opening mechanism is useful when a structure must be *tightly* grasped and retracted for a prolonged period of time. The spring causes the instrument to remain in a closed position, thereby obviating the need for exerting constant pressure on the handle by the surgeon or assistant.

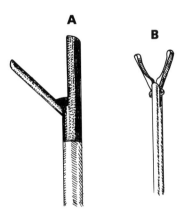

Fig. 8-13 **A,** Single- and **B,** double-action instrument tips.

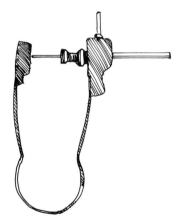

Fig. 8-14 Spring-loaded instrument handle for closing and opening the jaws of an instrument.

Another method to lock the tip of an instrument closed is by means of a built-in hand- (Fig. 8-15) or spring-operated ratchet. The ratchet mechanism can be used to place varying degrees of tension on the tissue that is grasped. Again, this may be useful for grasping a structure that needs to be lightly or tightly held and retracted.

Several tip designs are available for the grasping forceps. These can be divided into two broad categories: atraumatic and traumatic. *Atraumatic* graspers usually have serrated edges for the gentle manipulation of tissue. These are most often used for delicate grasping and dissection and come in a variety of tip shapes, including blunt, pointed (e.g., dolphin), straight (e.g., duck-bill), curved (e.g., Maryland), and angled (Fig. 8-16).

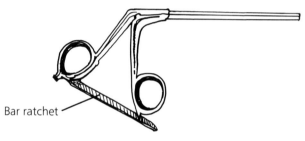

Fig. 8-15 Bar-type, hand-activated ratchet mechanism that is self-retaining for closing an instrument and locking the jaws in a "closed" position.

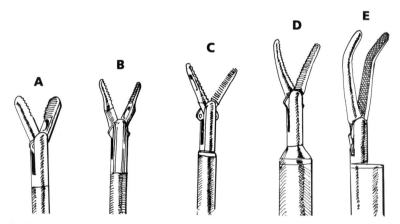

Fig. 8-16 Various types of grasping forceps configurations: **A,** Atraumatic blunt-coarse; **B,** atraumatic pointed (dolphin); **C,** atraumatic blunt-fine (duck-bill); **D,** atraumatic curved (Maryland); and **E,** atraumatic angled.

Traumatic graspers usually are toothed or clawed (Fig. 8-17, *A*). These instruments are used to grasp fibrous tissue tightly. They tend to have longer and broader jaws to facilitate grasping larger amounts of tissue in a secure fashion. Larger 11 mm spoon forceps are particularly helpful for retrieving biopsy specimens, gallstones, or smaller tissue specimens (e.g., pelvic lymph nodes) from the abdomen (Fig. 8-17, *B*).

More recently, newer laparoscopic graspers have been developed that duplicate other grasping instruments used during open surgical procedures. Several instrument companies have developed Allis, Babcock, and occlusive bowel clamps that can be used for specific laparoscopic purposes (Fig. 8-18). Moreover, instruments are now available with

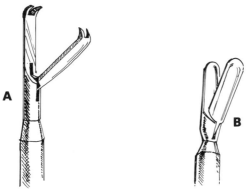

Fig. 8-17 A, Claw and **B,** spoon forceps for grasping and retrieving larger tissue specimens.

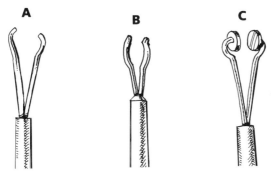

Fig. 8-18 Some special forceps for grasping tissue: **A,** Allis; **B,** Babcock; and **C,** bowel forceps.

both rotating and articulating tips to optimize access to the operative field and allow the surgeon to operate in a more comfortable position.

Incising instruments

An incision can be accomplished by endoscopic scissors, scalpel, electrosurgical probe, laser probe (CO_2), or a laser fiber (neodymium:yttrium aluminum garnet [Nd:YAG] or potassium titanyl phosphate [KTP]). Currently available laparoscopic *scissors* differ from their open surgical counterparts in that the blades are shorter and usually straight; as such, they cut a relatively smaller amount of tissue with each closure. Tips for the scissors are available in a variety of configurations: serrated tips for cutting fascia, curved pointed tips for dissection, and hooked tips for cutting suture material (Fig. 8-19, *A-C*). Many scissors are available with an electrosurgical connection to allow simultaneous electrocoagulation of the tissue as it is being mechanically cut. Other models of scissors are available with both rotating and angulating tips (Fig. 8-19, *D-F*).

Disposable and nondisposable scissors are available. The main difference between the two is that the nondisposable, reusable instruments tend to dull with time, thereby requiring sharpening at regular intervals. Presently a curved electrosurgical disposable type of scissors with a rotating shaft provides excellent access to the surgical site, allows for rapid dissection of tissue, provides for electrical incision and coagulation of tissue, and permits the surgeon to cut with mechanical (i.e., cold) shearing force when near the bowel or other delicate structures.

Laparoscopic *scalpel* blades are also available. They may be used to incise the common bile duct or to enter a fallopian tube at the site of an ectopic pregnancy. The surgeon must exercise great care while using these blades to prevent an inadvertent injury to the surrounding viscera.

Various types of *electrosurgical* instruments are available to incise or coagulate tissue (Fig. 8-20). Needle electrodes (e.g., Corson needle) are helpful to incise the peritoneum because they produce a very fine incision. Flat spatula electrodes are used to incise and bluntly dissect tissue. Hook (three-quarter circle and right-angle) electrodes can be passed beneath tissue to retract it away from more delicate neighboring structures before applying electrical current to incise the tissue. All of these instruments are insulated to prevent inadvertent leakage of current along the shaft. Many electrosurgical instruments also contain a suction/irrigation channel to suction smoke or fluid from the operative

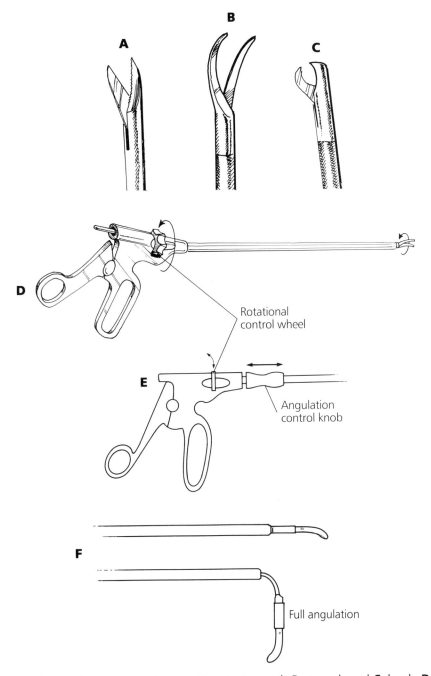

Fig. 8-19 Different types of scissor tips. **A,** Serrated; **B,** curved; and **C,** hook. **D,** In the rotating-curved scissors, by turning a wheel in the handle the scissors' tip can be rotated. **E** and **F,** In the rotating-angulating scissors, by pushing the angulation control knob down the shaft of the scissors, the scissors' tip can be made to angulate up to 90 degrees.

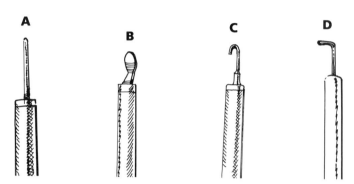

Fig. 8-20 Electrode tips. **A,** Corson; **B,** spatula; **C,** J hook; and **D,** right-angle or L hook.

field and to irrigate any area of bleeding in order to identify a bleeding vessel.

With the electrosurgical instruments, the usual settings for cutting and coagulation are in the 25 to 50 watt range. When using electrosurgical probes, the surgeon must be acutely aware of any other nearby instruments, because any unshielded metal portions of a juxtaposed grasper can conduct the electrical current if these graspers inadvertently come into contact with the activated electrosurgical probe. This explains, in part, the occurrence of bowel injuries distant from the site of surgery.

Also, care should be taken not to use a metal trocar sheath in combination with a plastic fixation sleeve; with this combination, any current transmitted to the metal trocar sheath will not be dissipated along the broad surface between the sheath and the abdominal wall, because the abdominal wall is insulated by the outer plastic fixation sleeve of the trocar. Therefore the current in the intra-abdominal portion of the metal sheath may build up considerably. If the bowel comes into contact with the metal portion of the trocar's sheath, a bowel injury may occur.

In addition, when using electrosurgery, the insulation of each instrument must be checked to ensure that there is no current leakage along the shaft of the instrument. *Also, the surgeon must constantly be aware that the entire bare metal portion of the cutting instrument is "live"; as such, the assistant operating the camera should be certain that the entire metal portion of the electrosurgical probe is in the field of view whenever the probe is activated.* Otherwise an unseen metal portion of the probe (e.g., a fixation screw) may contact and injure the bowel or other intra-abdominal structures.

The thickness of the instrument and the amount of exposed metal in contact with the tissue to be incised or coagulated are very important when using electrosurgical instruments. For cutting purposes, a thin metal tip provides the greatest current density and hence the most efficient cutting. The fine tip of these instruments can literally be activated and *gently stroked* along the tissue to be incised; it is not necessary to push the activated instrument firmly into the tissue to incise it. Indeed, cutting efficiency is greater when the electrode lies just off or gently touches the surface of the tissue to be incised.

Electrocoagulation is most efficiently done by using an insulated grasper to grasp the tissue to be coagulated and thereby appose both walls of the vessel. The coapted vessel is directly coagulated by sending current through the grasping forceps or indirectly coagulated by touching one side or the other of the tip of the insulated forceps with an activated electrosurgical probe in the coagulation mode. Again, in the latter situation, the entire exposed metal portion of both instruments must be clearly visible on the television monitor before any electrical current is applied.

Either monopolar or bipolar electrosurgical probes are available to the surgeon. The former is the most commonly available type of electrosurgical instrument; monopolar electrosurgery works with a remote ground (i.e., the "grounding" pad). As such, the current, once applied to the surgical site, then passes through the rest of the patient's body to the grounding pad. High energy levels are needed to accomplish a given cutting or hemostatic task. In contrast, with bipolar electrosurgery, the live and ground contacts are individually built into the tip of the instrument. Electrical current passes only between the two contacts. No grounding pad is used. Accordingly, less energy is needed to accomplish a task and the chance of inadvertent injury to surrounding structures is markedly decreased. Marked improvements in bipolar electrosurgical instrumentation have been made in recent years, and this mode of electrosurgery may eventually predominate.

Carbon dioxide (CO_2) lasers are also very commonly used in conjunction with laparoscopy. The CO_2 laser allows for precise cutting and excellent vaporization of surface lesions. It does not penetrate fluids and is not very efficient for cauterizing bleeding vessels. This laser modality is frequently used through the working channel of an operative laparoscope.

Both KTP (532 nm) and Nd:YAG (1064 nm) lasers may be delivered through fibers that are available in 400 μm and 600 μm size. Both lasers allow the surgeon to practice noncontact cutting and noncontact fulguration and vaporization of tissue. In addition, fibers with sculpted tips are available for more precise cutting with the KTP laser. The laser fibers are usually passed through an instrument such as an irrigator/aspirator for stabilization.

Table 8-1 lists the characteristics of lasers used with laparoscopy.

A filter is required between the laparoscope and the camera lens to prevent image distortion when the laser is fired. Also, if one is not using an attached video camera on the laparoscope, then an "in-line" filter system is necessary for eye protection. If a filter is not available, goggles with protective lenses must be worn by the entire operating room staff and by the patient when a KTP or an Nd:YAG laser is used, since the laser's wavelength is in the visible spectrum. Other precautions for avoiding eye injuries should be exercised according to the type of laser being used.

Retractors

Retractors are necessary to move and restrain overlying structures in order to provide direct access to the surgical site. The most basic retractor is a solid metal bar with a rounded atraumatic tip; this can be used to push back the bowel or the liver edge. More intricate retractors have recently been developed; some have several fingerlike projections housed within the shaft of the retractor. When extended, these blunt metal projections protrude from the tip of the instrument in a fanlike array, thereby providing a very wide retracting surface (Fig. 8-21). Similarly, other retractors have an intricate inner housing that allows them to be opened widely in the abdomen to act as a broad paddle for retraction purposes.

In addition, vein retractors are now available in 5 and 10 mm diameters for laparoscopic use. These may be useful in retracting the external iliac vein during pelvic lymph node dissection. Also, 14-gauge "needle" hook retractors are available; one or several of these can be separately introduced into the abdomen to retract tissue and provide proper exposure.

Table 8-1 Characteristics of lasers used for laparoscopic procedures

Laser type	Wavelength (μm)	Laser plume	Passes through fluids	Uses flexible fibers	Eye protection required	Special electrical hook-up	Cutting	Coagulation
CO_2	10.6	++++	0	No	Yes	No	++++	+
KTP	0.532	++	+++	Yes	Yes	Yes	+++	++
Nd:YAG	1.064	+	++++	Yes	Yes	Yes	+	++++

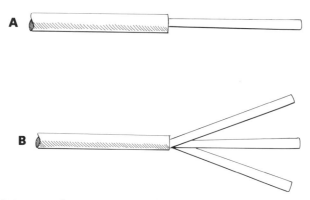

Fig. 8-21 Retractors: fan retractor, **A,** closed and **B,** open. This is useful for retracting bowel.

Uterine manipulators

Uterine manipulators are useful for increasing access to the bladder, adnexa, and cul-de-sac. Very simple instruments that provide uterine elevation include cervical dilators or instruments placed on the cervix, such as a tenaculum. These provide suboptimal movement, and their use is quite limited. In contrast, the Hulka clamp is a simply designed instrument that will provide adequate uterine manipulation for most cases. This is placed following steps that are appropriate for most uterine manipulators. A pelvic examination is performed after bladder drainage to determine the location of the uterine fundus. An open-sided bivalve speculum is then inserted and the anterior lip of the cervix is grasped with a single-tooth tenaculum. It is important to grasp the cervix well but not to injure the bladder. While stabilizing the cervix the protrusion from the Hulka clamp is placed into the cervix, and the anterior lip of the cervix is grasped by the tooth of the clamp. The tenaculum and speculum are then removed, because leaving them in would hamper movement of the uterus. The posterior forchette is protected by placing a moistened 4 × 4 gauze pad into the vagina posterior to the clamp.

More sophisticated manipulators also allow dye instillation for assessment of fallopian tube patency (Fig. 8-22). Two commonly used instruments are the Cohen-Eder and the Valtchev manipulators. Both

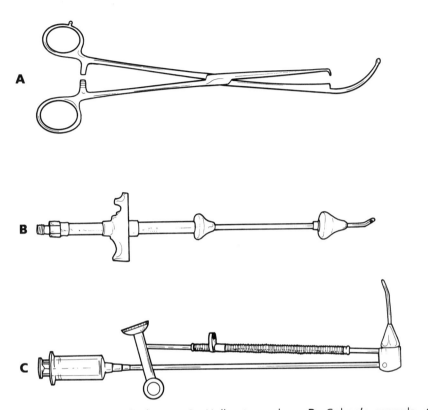

Fig. 8-22 Uterine manipulators: **A,** Hulka tenaculum. **B,** Cohen's cannula. **C,** Valtchev uterine mobilizer.

are reusable and are held in place by a tenaculum that is attached to the cervix. The Cohen-Eder device features various sizes of cannula (acorn) tips that may be attached pointing forward or backward, depending on the orientation of the uterus (anteverted or retroverted). The Valtchev manipulator (Fig. 8-23) has two similar cannulas as well as four interchangeable obturators to accommodate various clinical situations. The Valtchev instrument's design makes it possible to be released, and then locked again into the desired position (Fig. 8-23, *A* and *B*). With either instrument, dye instillation is accomplished by attaching a syringe to the Luer Lock's external end and pulsing dye

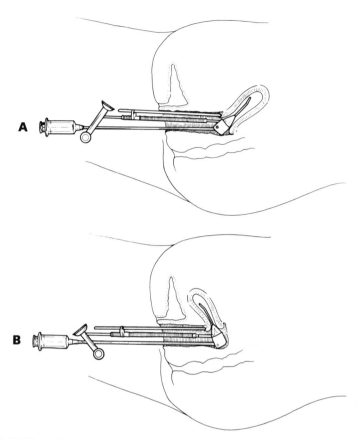

Fig. 8-23 The Valtchev uterine mobilizer: **A,** The tip of the mobilizer is in the uterine cavity. **B,** By rotating the spacer arm counterclockwise, the head, with attached obturator and cannula, anteverts the uterus.

into the uterine cavity. Alternatively, IV extension tubing may be placed between the dye source and the syringe so that the surgeon or assistant may control dye passage from the sterile field. Instillation is usually performed with dilute methylene blue, which is readily discernible from the intra-abdominal irrigant.

Also available are a number of disposable instruments for both manipulation and dye instillation (Fig. 8-24). Typically these are held in place by intrauterine balloons. When using these instruments to estab-

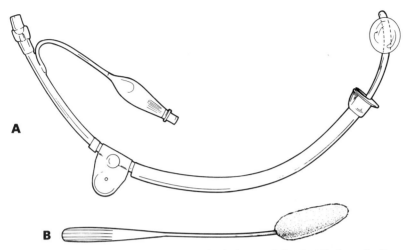

Fig. 8-24 Disposable instruments for manipulation and dye instillation: **A,** Kronner Manipujector. **B,** Rectal probe.

lish tubal patency, one must use care to avoid overdistention of the balloons, which may occlude the tubal ostia. Some of these products also feature a second balloon that inflates against the external cervical os and prevents backflow of contrast material. Manipulation with these products is usually inferior to that with reusable instruments.

Whenever working laparoscopically in the true pelvis on a female patient, one will likely benefit from use of a uterine manipulator. At times rectal probes may also provide better access or definition of anatomy. For example, when the cul-de-sac is involved with endometriosis or adhesive disease and the location of the rectum is unclear, the surgical assistant may effectively retract the rectum with a rectal probe. If probes are not available, a digital examination will at least help define the anatomy.

As with any surgical instrument, uterine manipulators should be used appropriately and with care. The individual moving the instrument must understand that the movement of the uterus is opposite to that of the manipulator; thus to elevate the uterus one must push downward on the manipulator. Improper placement or handling of these instruments can result in uterine perforation. Also, care must be taken not to traumatize the vaginal wall. In addition, cervical manipulation may result in a vagal reaction and marked bradycardia. In general these instruments are not used for pregnant patients.

Needle holders

Several types of laparoscopic needle holders are available. The handles are of a locking design to hold the needle tightly in place; this is usually accomplished with a spring-loaded or ratchet mechanism.

There are two basic types of tips on needle holders: a hinged jaw or a sliding sheath. The hinged jaw needle holders usually have one jaw fixed (i.e., single action) so the needle can be more easily positioned in the jaws prior to intracorporeal suturing (Fig. 8-25). Some hinged jaw needle drivers contain a notch at the inner portion of the hinge in which the needle can be seated firmly to reduce needle rotation. The hinged jaws usually are controlled by a routine scissors-type handle containing a ratchet locking mechanism. Recent modifications of this type of needle holder include diamond-jaw-V surfaces for a more secure grasp of the needle; coaxial, in-line handles; and Castro-Viejo locking mechanisms.

In contrast, the sliding sheath needle holders consist of a cylindrical tube with a distal notch for needle positioning (Fig. 8-26). The needle is held in position by an inner spring-loaded sliding sheath. When "at rest," each of the three different needle holders holds the needle in only one of three directions: 45 degrees right, 45 degrees left, or 90 degrees to the shaft of the needle holder. The needle holders are opened by squeezing the handle. If the needle's shaft is edged in its design, only one position of the needle is possible once the handle has been released. As such, the needle becomes automatically seated in the correct alignment.

Knot pushers

Knot pushers are available to aid delivery of knots tied extracorporeally (Fig. 8-27). The reusable knot pushers are basically metal bars with a notch cut in the end. A throw of the suture is created extracorporeally and then by threading the suture across the open prongs of the knot pusher, the knot can be pushed downward through the trocar sheath and delivered across the peritoneal cavity to the surgical site.

Tissue removal

Some tissue specimens (e.g., appendix, ovary, gallbladder, lymph nodes) may be removed directly through the ≥10 mm laparoscopic sheath; larger tissue specimens (e.g., kidney, spleen, kidney plus ureter) may need to be entrapped and morcellated before removal.

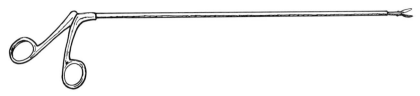

Fig. 8-25 Hinged jaw type of needle holder.

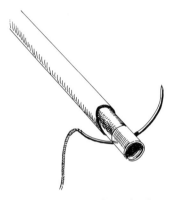

Fig. 8-26 Sliding sheath type of needle holder. The inner sliding sheath is spring-loaded; this maintains appropriate orientation of the needle and holds it firmly in position.

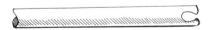

Fig. 8-27 Knot pusher has a notch at its tip, which is used to slide an extracorporeally formed "throw" (i.e., half hitch) through the laparoscope sheath and down onto tissue within the peritoneal cavity.

Laparoscopic *entrapment sacks* are made of either a durable double layer of impenetrable nylon and plastic or a single layer of thick-walled plastic (Appendix A-6). The sacks are impermeable to bacteria and tissue and contain a proximal closure mechanism. The closure mechanism may be a drawstring which not only closes the neck of the sack but also serves as a handle to pull the sack up through a ≥10 mm trocar site (Fig. 8-28). Alternatively, a drawstring may be loaded through a plastic rod, which the surgeon can use to help pull the sack through the trocar site, or the closure mechanism may be a band of spring metal that causes the mouth of the sack to automatically open when it is introduced into the abdomen and to close as it is withdrawn from the abdomen.

If the specimen is too large to deliver intact, then after the neck of the sack is delivered onto the abdominal wall, a morcellator or a forceps (e.g., ring forceps or Kelly clamp) is necessary to fragment and remove the tissue from the sack, after which the empty sack can be pulled from the abdominal cavity. The fragmentation procedure is monitored laparoscopically so that if the sack is perforated, the perforation is immediately noted. At this point the trocar site would be incised and the torn sack and its contents could be extracted intact. For morcellation purposes, the sack constructed of nylon and plastic is preferable.

Morcellation devices of the tissue punch variety were designed for gynecologic use (Fig. 8-29). These 10 mm instruments take "bites" of tissue using a scissors-type handle mechanism. The pieces of tissue are sequentially transported up the shaft of the instrument as each bite of tissue is taken. When using this instrument, the tissue to be removed is not placed in an entrapment sack.

Clinical trials have begun with a laparoscopic cavitron ultrasonic aspirator (CUSA). This device can morcellate and aspirate soft tissue and may be a useful adjunct in lymph node dissections. To use this device, the tissue does not need to be entrapped.

Other morcellators fragment tissue with an electrically powered (4000 to 5000 rpm) cylindrical blade recessed in a 10 mm metal sheath that has an atraumatic tip (Fig. 8-30). The blade rapidly slices any tissue cored into the morcellator's sheath; the fragments of tissue are aspirated into a wire mesh trap located in the handle of the morcellator. This type of morcellator removes tissue quickly and efficiently. *However, the electric morcellator must always be used in conjunction with the plastic and nylon laparoscopic entrapment sack to avoid injury to any surrounding tissues.* If an electrical aspirating morcellator is being used, any perforation of the sack will cause an immediate loss of the pneumoperitoneum. Accordingly, the entire morcellation process must be endoscopically monitored.

When the specimen is entrapped in a plastic and nylon entrapment sack, morcellation can be accomplished quite simply with a blunt Kelly clamp and a ring forceps. These instruments can be sequentially introduced into the sack, and the entrapped tissue can be fragmented and manually removed bit by bit. Although lacking in elegance, this method is safe, effective, inexpensive, and readily available.

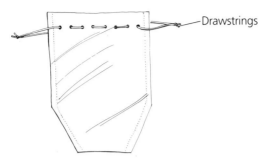

Fig. 8-28 Tissue entrapment sack: nylon and plastic construction. Once the tissue is placed within the sack in the peritoneal cavity, the neck of the sack is closed by pulling on the drawstrings. The neck of the sack is then withdrawn through a ≥10 mm trocar site. (Shown: a 2- × 5-inch sack.)

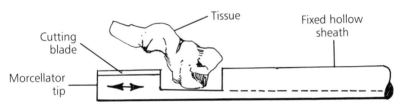

Fig. 8-29 Hand-held punch type of tissue morcellator. Cores of tissue are stored within the hollow sheath as the tissue is fragmented.

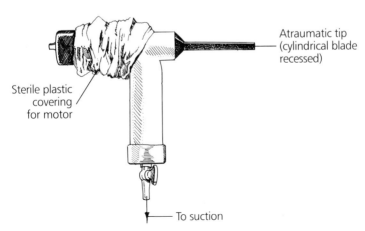

Fig. 8-30 With the electrical tissue morcellator, a cylindrical recessed blade cuts tissue that is cored into the outer atraumatic sheath. The fragmented tissue is then aspirated through the sheath and stored within a wire mesh trap in the handle.

ASPIRATION/IRRIGATION SYSTEMS

There are both aspiration and combined aspiration/irrigation devices available. The latter are preferable. The aspirating channel may be attached directly to an OR vacuum/collection system. Most aspirating channels consist of a simple metal tube with either a one-way stopcock or spring-controlled trumpet valve (Fig. 8-31) to regulate the suction; the latter is preferable because it is easier to use. They are available in diameters ranging from 5 to 10 mm in both disposable and reusable models. The suction tip may have a single opening or several smaller holes (i.e., pool suction) along the distal shaft. The problem with most aspiration units presently available is their small diameter; as such, the holes of the aspirator have a tendency to obstruct with tissue or fat.

The irrigation channel is controlled with a one-way stopcock or trumpet valve (see Fig. 8-31); again, the latter type is preferable. Gravity flow is usually insufficient to clear clots; therefore pressurizing the irrigant (250 to 700 mm Hg) is recommended. A blood pressure cuff or purpose-designed pressure bag may be placed around the irrigant bag, and the pressure can thus be raised to 250 mm Hg. Alternatively, a CO_2-driven device (Nezhat) is available that pressurizes the irrigant up to 700 mm Hg (Fig. 8-32). At this higher pressure, the flow of irrigant can be used for blunt dissection; adhesions can be better defined and fatty tissue can be displaced. This technique of dissection is known as aquadissection or hydrodissection.

The irrigation fluid that is most commonly used is saline or lactated Ringer's solution. Heparin (5000 U/L) may be added to prevent the formation of blood clots, which are difficult to aspirate once formed. Also, a broad-spectrum antibiotic (e.g., 500 mg cefazolin/L) may be added to the first 1 or 2 L of irrigant.

MISCELLANEOUS INSTRUMENTS

Several other instruments are available for specific uses. Laparoscopic Doppler probes as small as 5 mm can be used to detect blood vessels. This instrument may be useful in identifying the testicular artery during laparoscopic varix ligation or for identifying the renal artery during a laparoscopic nephrectomy.

A long-needle aspirating probe is available. (See Appendix A-7 for more information.) A Luer Lock hub is attached to the handle of this device. This needle can be useful for decompressing a hydropic gallbladder, draining an ovarian cyst, or confirming the location of a renal cyst or lymphocele.

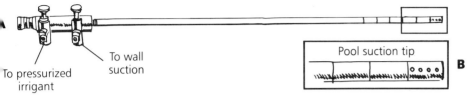

Fig. 8-31 A, Combined aspiration/irrigation instrument has a trumpet valve mechanism for separately activating suction and irrigation. **B,** Inset, pool suction tip.

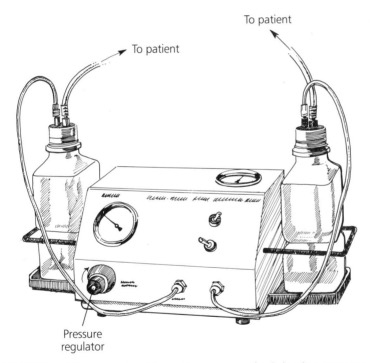

Fig. 8-32 With a CO_2-pressurized/irrigation system, the irrigation pressure can be preset up to 700 mm Hg. The higher pressure can be used to aid tissue dissection (i.e., hydrodissection). The return line from the patient is connected to wall suction. This system is typically attached to an instrument similar to the one shown in Fig. 8-31 or to one of several other reusable attachments that are available in both 5 and 10 mm sizes.

The argon beam coagulator can be used for laparoscopic work. Five and 10 mm probes are available. The argon beam coagulator uses argon gas (at 4 L/min flow) to clear the surgical field and to deliver electrical current to a bleeding surface, thereby electrofulgurating the tissue. The probe never comes into direct contact with the tissue. The surface temperature of the fulgurated tissue remains at just under 100° C, and the depth of injury is only 1 to 2 mm (versus 5 mm with standard electrocautery). This instrument is helpful during laparoscopic, hepatic, splenic, or renal surgery; parenchymal surfaces and vessels ≤4 mm can be effectively fulgurated.

INSTRUMENT PASSAGE

Instruments of 5 mm can be passed directly into the 5 mm sheath. If a 10, 11, or 12 mm sheath is in place, a 5.5 mm or preferably a 4.5 mm reducer must be affixed to the top of the sheath before passage of the 5 mm instrument (Fig. 8-33). In passing the instrument, the sheath should be steadied with the nondominant hand or by the assistant so that it is not inadvertently pushed deeper into the abdominal cavity and to facilitate instrument entry into the sheath. Likewise, when ex-

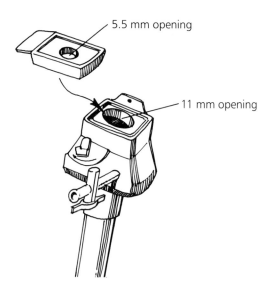

5.5 mm opening

11 mm opening

Fig. 8-33 A 5.5 mm reducer being placed onto an 11 mm sheath in preparation for passage of a 5 mm instrument.

changing instruments, it is helpful if the assistant stabilizes the sheath while the surgeon steadies and passes the next instrument into the sheath.

Each instrument must be monitored as it enters the abdomen. As such, the laparoscope should be focused on the end of the sheath through which the *closed* instrument is being passed so as to "watch" it enter the abdomen (Fig. 8-34). Blind passage of instruments into the abdomen can result in significant, and at times unrecognized, injury

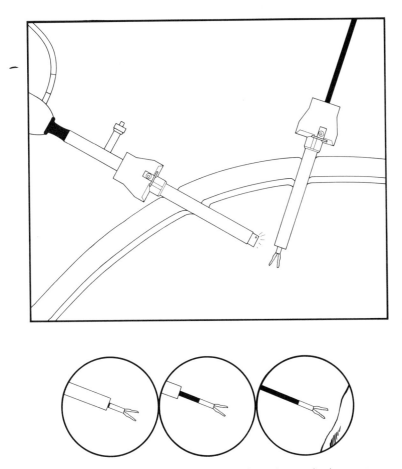

Fig. 8-34 Laparoscopic monitoring of instrument insertion and advancement to the surgical site.

to the underlying viscera (Fig. 8-35). Also, all grasping instruments should be passed with their jaws closed; the jaws should only be opened at the surgical site under endoscopic control. ("Don't open your mouth unless you have something to say.")

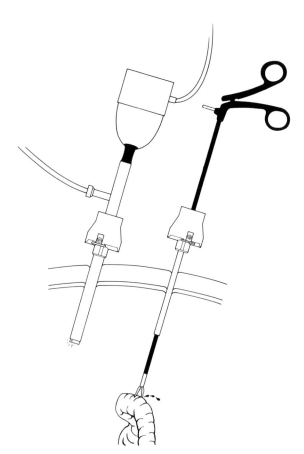

Fig. 8-35 Bowel injury caused by unmonitored passage of a pointed, inadvertently opened grasper into the abdominal cavity.

LAPAROTOMY SET

In addition to the laparoscopic equipment, a full laparotomy set should be available in the event that emergent exploration is required. This table should be in the laparoscopy room so that the abdomen can be opened at a moment's notice if a vascular catastrophe occurs during the laparoscopic procedure. Also, during routine laparoscopy many open-type instruments should be on the table: a knife handle with a blade (No. 11, 12, or 15), suture scissors, towel clips, Kelly clamps, straight mosquito clamps, ring forceps, needle drivers, retractors (e.g., Army/Navy, Sinn), and fascial clamps (e.g., Allis, Kocher).

TROUBLESHOOTING

Problem: Air leak around the instrument.
Solution: Use a 4.5 mm reducer on the 5 mm sheath to create a tighter seal.

Problem: Inadvertent removal of the trocar sheath (or "I should have sewn it in *!!*").
Solution:

- Focus the laparoscope on the peritoneotomy site. Load the obturator so that it is rotated 180 degrees, thereby preventing it from being properly seated on the sheath. The safety shield will thus remain in an extended, locked position. As such, the sharp obturator will not be exposed while trying to reenter the initial peritoneotomy site, thereby precluding a second peritoneotomy. Slide the trocar back into the abdomen through the original peritoneotomy, remove the obturator, and sew the sheath to the skin with a No. 2 nonabsorbable suture to avoid its inadvertent removal again (Fig. 8-36).
- Backload the trocar sheath on a blunt-tipped grasping forceps, and under endoscopic control the tip of the forceps can be passed through the skin site and guided until it traverses the peritoneotomy. The trocar sheath can then be slid over the instrument until the sheath is in the abdomen; the instrument is then removed, and the sheath is affixed to the skin with a No. 2 nonabsorbable suture (Fig. 8-37).

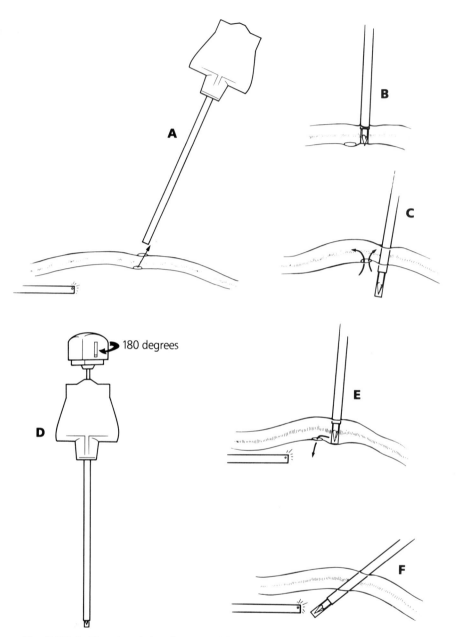

Fig. 8-36 A, The sheath has been accidentally pulled from the abdominal cavity. **B** and **C,** If the sharp obturator is replaced in the sheath, then a separate, new peritoneotomy may be made. Thus gas may leak through the original peritoneotomy, resulting in significant insufflation of the properitoneal and subcutaneous space. **D,** If the sharp obturator is replaced but rotated 180 degrees, it will not seat properly within the sheath; hence the safety shield on the obturator will *not* retract. **E** and **F,** The blunt tip of the obturator can be endoscopically guided to the original peritoneotomy site. The sheath is now secured to the skin with a No. 2 nonabsorbable suture.

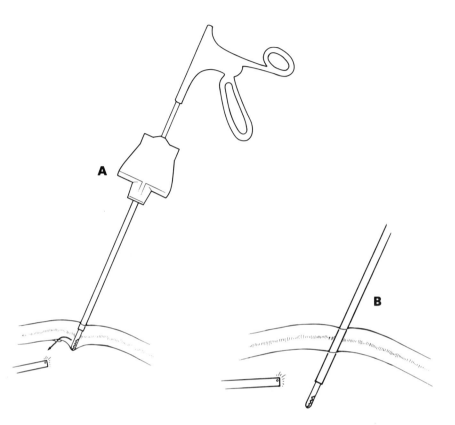

Fig. 8-37 A, When a sheath has been inadvertently removed from the abdomen, the surgeon can *backload* the sheath on a blunt-tipped laparoscopic grasping forceps. The *closed* forceps is passed through the skin site and **B,** is maneuvered until it enters the abdomen through the original peritoneotomy site. The sheath is then slid forward along the shaft of the forceps until the tip of the laparoscopic sheath lies well within the abdominal cavity. The sheath is now secured to the skin with a No. 2 nonabsorbable suture and the grasping forceps is removed.

REFERENCES

1. Kavoussi LR, Clayman RV. Trocar fixation during laparoscopy. J Endourology 6:71, 1992.
2. Semm K. Instruments and equipment for endoscopic abdominal surgery. In Operative Manual for Endoscopic Abdominal Surgery. Chicago: Year Book, 1987, pp 46-124.
3. Talamini MA, Gadacz TR. Laparoscopic equipment and instrumentation. In Zucker KA (ed). Surgical Laparoscopy. St. Louis: Quality Medical Publishing, Inc, 1991, pp 23-77.
4. ACOG Technical Bulletin. Laser Technology. No. 146, Sept 1990.

CHAPTER 9

Laparoscopic Suturing and Knot Tying

Elspeth M. McDougall and Nathaniel J. Soper

One of the more challenging aspects of laparoscopic surgery is knot tying. This skill enables the surgeon to ligate vessels, reapproximate tissue surfaces, and reconstruct organs as he or she does at open surgery. As such, mastery of suturing techniques greatly enhances the surgeon's ability to enter the realm of therapeutic laparoscopy. This chapter will summarize each of the knot-tying techniques currently available.

EQUIPMENT LIST

1. *Laparoscopic trocars* used during suturing vary from 5 to 12 mm in diameter; either disposable or reusable trocars may be used.

2. *Reducer caps* allow working instruments of smaller diameter (i.e., 3.5 to 10.5 mm) to be used through larger laparoscopic ports (i.e., 5 to 12 mm) without the loss of the pneumoperitoneum. These plastic caps are readily affixed to the top of the laparoscopic cannula.

3. *Laparoscopic 5 mm needle holders* are used to grasp and manipulate needles during laparoscopic suturing. These needle holders may be single or double action. The single-action needle holder has one fixed jaw and a single movable jaw; both jaws are movable in the double-action needle holder. The jaws may have a diamond-pattern texture to provide a more secure grip on the needle. A jaw-opening mechanism has recently been developed that lies entirely flush with the shaft of the instrument during opening and closing of the jaws. This design greatly facilitates intracorporeal knot tying because any pre-formed loops of suture made on the shaft of the needle holder can be easily slid or pushed off the shaft of these instruments without getting caught in the mechanism.

   Alternatively, a spring-operated needle holder with straight or fixed angles (45 degrees right, 45 degrees left, or 90 degrees) may be used (Fig. 9-1, *A*). Once the needle is grasped, it is automatically held tightly in the jaw of the forceps at the predetermined angle inherent in the needle holder's jaw (Fig. 9-1, *B*). A Castro-Viejo type of locking mechanism has recently been designed into a laparoscopic

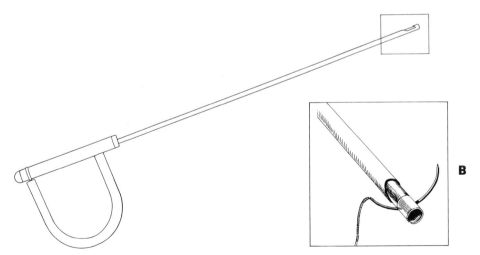

Fig. 9-1 A, Spring-operated needle holder. **B,** Needle properly seated.

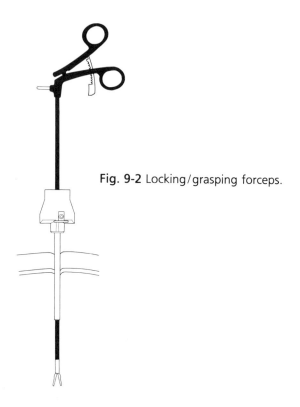

Fig. 9-2 Locking/grasping forceps.

needle holder; this mechanism facilitates the opening and closing of the jaws of the needle holder from any rotational position. Needle holders with this locking mechanism also have handles that are aligned coaxially with the shaft rather than arising at right angles. This feature facilitates rotational movements of the instrument's tip.
4. *Tissue graspers* are usually 5 mm in diameter and are helpful to grasp the tissue to be sewn, to grasp the tail end of the suture, and to assist in the proper positioning of the needle within the jaws of the needle holder. A *locking* atraumatic type of grasper is preferred (Fig. 9-2). For "following" a running suture, a rubber-shod grasper is recommended to preclude any damage to the suture material.
5. *Suture introducers* are capped metal cylinder inserts that are the same length but of smaller diameter than the trocar sheath; they facilitate the smooth introduction of ligatures, sutures, and 5 mm instruments through the 11 or 12 mm trocar ports (Fig. 9-3).
6. *Hook scissors* are used for cutting the suture material.

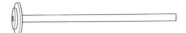

Fig. 9-3 Suture introducer.

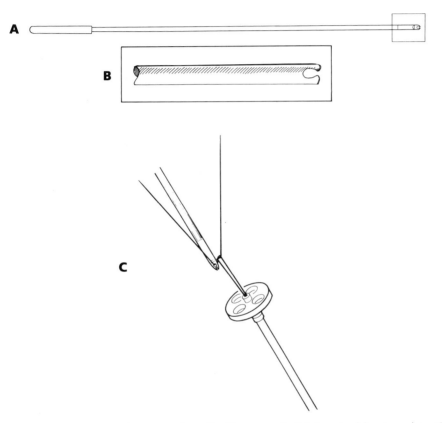

Fig. 9-4 **A,** Knot pusher, overview. **B,** Close-up of distal end of knot pusher. **C,** Knot pusher being used to deliver the first throw of a knot into the suture introducer.

7. *Knot pushers,* either independent or integral with the suture material itself, facilitate delivery of extracorporeally tied knots into the abdomen. The independent knot pusher is used to simply slide (Clarke-Riech) (Fig. 9-4) or slide and cinch (Gazayerli) (Fig. 9-5) the knot into place. The integral type of knot pusher is attached to a preformed knotted loop in the suture; after the loop is passed over the tissue to be secured, the integral plastic knot pusher is snapped free from

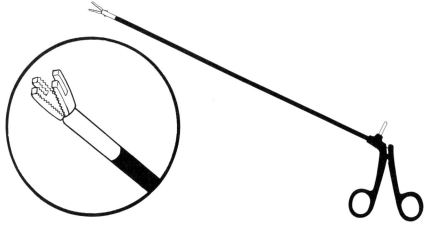

Fig. 9-5 Gazayerli knot pusher.

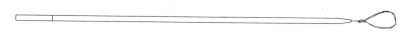

Fig. 9-6 Ligature loop.

its terminal plastic base and used to deliver and secure the preformed knot (Fig. 9-6).

SUTURING: CONCEPTS

For laparoscopic sewing a small amount of forethought can save the surgeon much intraoperative frustration and time. First, the surgeon will need three ≥10 mm ports through which to sew. While smaller 5 mm ports can be used, this limits the surgeon's options and the size of the needle that can be used.

The three ports must be arranged so that the laparoscopic port is flanked and behind the two "suturing" ports (Fig. 9-7). This should result in a situation whereby the tips of the two suturing ports and the tip of the endoscopic port each enter the surgical field at oblique angles to one another. Also, each port should be at least 2 inches away from any other port. This should eliminate the problems of crossed sheaths (i.e., "crossing swords") inside the patient or the difficulty of having the trocar sheaths too close together (i.e., "striking handles") outside the patient. Finally, when placing the trocars, it is helpful to have them close enough to the operative site to permit access with no more than

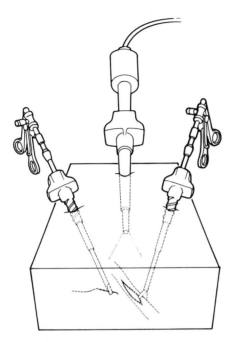

Fig. 9-7 Correct arrangement of laparoscopic ports for suturing. Laparoscope is behind and between suturing instruments, which enter operative field from oblique angles.

half the shaft length (i.e., 30 cm) of the standard needle holder or grasper.

If the ports are placed in the previously described manner, the instruments will enter the field of view tangentially and not coaxially. This will afford the surgeon a modicum of depth perception and will prevent the instrument from blocking the surgeon's view of the operative site. Furthermore, with this trocar arrangement, the instrument should always be moving away from the laparoscope, thereby avoiding any "mirror image" situations.

When one is suturing, the video monitor should be in line with the surgeon and the operative field. The surgeon must continually view the screen; time spent looking at one's hands is time wasted.

Laparoscopic suturing is a learned skill, not an innate talent. Practice and continuous experience are essential to mastering these advanced techniques. Because the image is magnified many times, each movement must be slowed accordingly; therefore, each motion must be precise and efficient to avoid retarding the procedure excessively.

SUTURE PLACEMENT
Preformed ligature loop

The preformed ligature loop is useful in ligating a divided vascular pedicle (e.g., ovarian), the stump of a blood vessel, or the appendix (see Fig. 9-6).

Instrumentation   Ligature loop (0 plain, 0 chromic, or PDS), 10 mm suture introducer sheath, 5 mm locking atraumatic grasper, 5 mm reducer cap, 10.5 mm reducer cap, and hook scissors.

Technique

1. *Backload* the plastic shaft of the preformed ligature loop through a 10 mm introducer sheath (see Fig. 9-3).
2. Retract the plastic shaft through the 10 mm introducer sheath (Fig. 9-8, *A*) until the knot and loop reside completely inside the 10 mm introducer sheath.
3. Place the 10.5 mm reducer cap onto the 11 or 12 mm laparoscopic sheath.
4. Insert the 10 mm introducer into the 11 or 12 mm trocar port, which is now overlaid with a 10.5 mm reducer cap (Fig. 9-8, *B*). Advance the introducer until it abuts the reducer cap (Fig. 9-8, *C*).

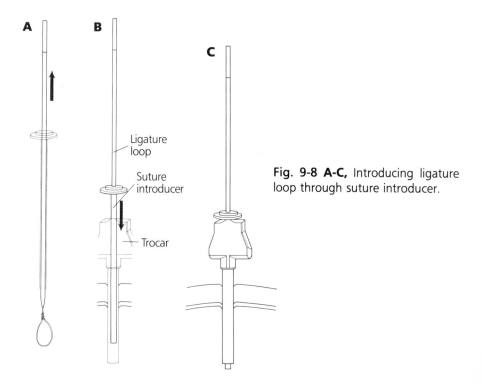

A   **B**   **C**

Ligature loop

Suture introducer

Trocar

Fig. 9-8 A-C, Introducing ligature loop through suture introducer.

5. Advance the plastic shaft of the ligature loop through the 10 mm introducer until the loop is completely exposed inside the abdomen (Fig. 9-9).
6. Insert a 5 mm grasper through a separate laparoscopic sheath. If the sheath is ≥10 mm, place a 5 mm reducer cap. Pass the tip of the 5 mm grasper through the loop of the ligature.
7. Grasp the targeted tissue pedicle with the same 5 mm grasper and lock the jaws. Maneuver the loop downward until it goes beyond the tip of the grasper and encircles the targeted tissue.
8. Alternatively, the grasped tissue can be pulled upward through the loop (Fig. 9-10).
9. To tighten the ligature loop, the surgeon snaps the shaft at the red band, thereby cracking the shaft into two pieces, one short (proximal) and one long (distal) (Fig. 9-11). Pull upward simultaneously

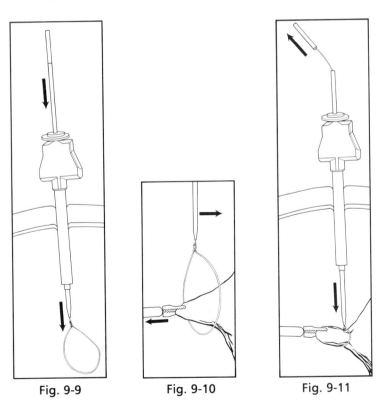

Fig. 9-9   Fig. 9-10   Fig. 9-11

Fig. 9-9 Ligature loop fully introduced into abdominal cavity.
Fig. 9-10 Tissue grasped and pulled through ligature loop.
Fig. 9-11 Ligature loop cinched down tightly.

on the small proximal end of the shaft and slide the long distal portion of the plastic shaft downward. This slides the knot forward and causes the loop to decrease in size as it tightens around the tissue. During this maneuver the 5 mm grasper, now held by the assistant, must keep the tissue steady, while upward traction on the tissue is exerted through the loop ligature by pulling upward on the proximal (short) end of the plastic shaft.

10. Holding the tissue in the grasper and simultaneously tightening the ligature loop beneath the grasper allows precise placement of the ligature.

11. After snugging the ligature loop onto the tissue, the tissue is released from the grasper. Additional tightening of the ligature knot, for maximal hemostasis, is achieved by a two-handed maneuver. While steadying the short proximal end portion of the plastic shaft of the ligature loop with one hand, the other hand pushes firmly on the long distal portion of the plastic shaft of the loop ligature to cinch the knot. This maneuver is repeated three times. Once the knot is locked down securely, the plastic distal shaft of the ligature loop is drawn up into the introducer away from the knot.

12. The 5 mm grasper is withdrawn and replaced with a 5 mm hook scissors. The suture is cut, leaving a ¼-inch tail (Fig. 9-12). If the 5 mm grasper must remain on the tissue for the knot to be properly visualized, then the hook scissors can be introduced through the same trocar through which the loop ligature was passed. To do

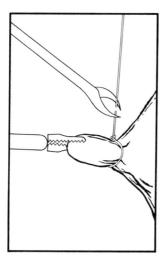

Fig. 9-12 Suture cut with scissors.

this, the suture must first be cut at the level of the short proximal end of the plastic rod; then the short proximal end and long distal portion of the loop plastic rod (i.e., the knot pusher) can be removed. Pass the end of the now-bare suture through a 5 mm reducer and affix the reducer onto the 11 or 12 mm port; the 5 mm hook scissors are inserted through the 5 mm reducer alongside the suture and are used to cut the suture, leaving a ¼-inch tail.

Free tie

This technique is particularly suitable for securing an uncut vessel.

Instrumentation   A 5 mm needle holder, 5 or 10 mm curved grasping forceps, 10 mm suture introducer, 5 mm hook scissors, knot pusher, 36 inches of suture material (no needle), and a 10.5 mm reducer cap.

Technique

1. Grasp the suture at one end with the 5 mm needle holder so that 1 inch of suture material lies beyond the jaws of the needle holder. Put a mosquito clamp on the opposite end of the suture so it cannot be inadvertently pulled into the 10 mm introducer.
2. Insert the introducer with the 1-inch protruding tail of suture into the 10 mm suture introducer cannula (Fig. 9-13).
3. Advance the loaded 10 mm suture introducer through the 11 or 12 mm trocar port after affixing the 10.5 mm reducer cap.
4. Insert 5 or 10 mm curved tissue-grasping forceps through another trocar port.
5. Position the curved grasping forceps so that the tip of the jaws traverse the backside of the vessel.
6. Move the needle holder deeper into the abdomen until the 1-inch protruding tail of the suture just proximal to the jaws of the needle holder can be grasped by the forceps.
7. Open the needle holder and release the suture.
8. Withdraw the needle holder to the tip of the suture introducer and use it to grasp the suture material where it enters the abdomen at the end of the 10 mm suture introducer.
9. Reinsert the needle holder to the site of the vessel, thereby bringing approximately 6 inches of suture material into the abdomen.
10. Gently move the curved grasping forceps upward until the suture encircles the vessel (Fig. 9-14).
11. Regrasp the tail of the suture with the needle holder (Fig. 9-15).
12. Use the curved grasping forceps to help guide the suture around the vessel so there is no tension or "sawing" of the vessel as the

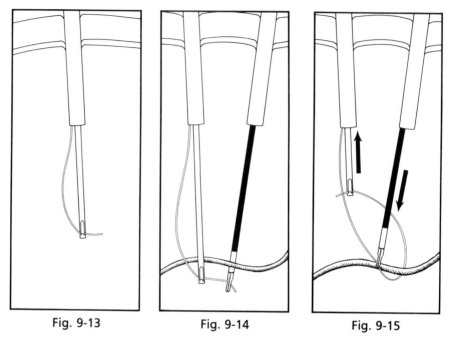

Fig. 9-13   Fig. 9-14   Fig. 9-15

Fig. 9-13 Free suture passed through trocar.
Fig. 9-14 Grasper pulls end of suture around vessel.
Fig. 9-15 Needle holder pulls suture end into trocar and onto the abdominal wall.
The grasper is used to guide the suture around the tissue so there is no "sawing."

needle holder pulls the tail of the suture into and through the 10 mm suture introducer.

13. The assistant now covers the introducer channel with a finger to prevent loss of the pneumoperitoneum. The needle holder is opened, thereby releasing its grasp on the suture now that both ends lie outside the 10 mm suture introducer. The needle holder can now be removed from the table. An extracorporeal square knot or locking loop knot can now be tied.

"Stick tie"—straight needle

This technique is excellent for sewing the stump of the appendix closed or closing a small enterotomy or cystotomy.

Instrumentation A 5 mm needle holder, 5 mm locking atraumatic grasping forceps, 10 mm suture introducer, 5 mm hook scissors, 36 inches of suture on a straight or curved (T-31) taper needle (19 mm), 10.5 mm reducer cap, and knot pusher. Alternatively, a preformed kit may be used in which the needle, suture, and knot pusher come as an integrated unit.

Technique
1. With the 5 mm needle holder, grasp the *suture* above its junction with the straight needle so that the needle will lie flat against the shaft of the needle holder. Insert the 5 mm needle holder with the needle/suture into the 10 mm suture introducer cannula. Alternatively, if a curved needle is being used, pass the grasper through the 10 mm suture introducer, grasp the suture just above its junction with the needle, and pull the curved needle lengthwise into the introducer.
2. Affix the 10.5 mm reducer cap to the 11 or 12 mm trocar sheath. Advance the loaded 10 mm suture introducer through the 11 or 12 mm sheath.
3. Insert 5 mm tissue-grasping forceps through another trocar port.
4. Advance the needle holder into the abdominal cavity. Use the 5 mm grasping forceps to grasp the needle, which should now be dangling from the needle holder.
5. Open the needle holder, thereby releasing the suture. Now use the needle holder to grasp the shaft of the needle at a right angle to the needle. Use the grasping forceps to help steady the needle until it rests securely within the jaws of the needle holder. The 5 mm grasping forceps is then opened, thereby releasing the needle to the needle holder.
6. Use the 5 mm grasping forceps to depress or grasp and hold taut the tissue to be sewn. Pass the needle through the tissue with the needle holder until the tip of the needle exits the tissue opposite the point of entry (Fig. 9-16).
7. While maintaining the position of the needle holder (thereby continuing to immobilize the pierced tissue), use the 5 mm grasping forceps to grasp the needle tip as it exits the tissue. Pull the needle through the tissue. If an additional pass of the needle is required (e.g., Z stitch or "figure-of-eight" stitch), steps 6 through 8 are repeated. Now the needle holder is used to grasp the suture material directly behind the needle again.

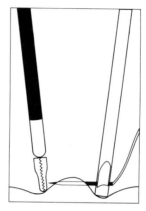

Fig. 9-16 Needle passed through tissue; the tissue is steadied by the 5 mm grasper.

8. With the 5 mm grasping forceps, pull additional suture length into the abdominal cavity to minimize tension on the tissue from the suture.

9. Use the 5 mm grasping forceps to draw the extra suture material through the tissue in the direction of the needle's path.

10. The needle holder, still holding the suture just below the needle/suture junction, is withdrawn completely through the 10 mm suture introducer. There should be little or no tension on the sewn tissue as this is done.

11. The assistant covers the introducer channel with a finger to prevent loss of pneumoperitoneum. The surgeon cuts the needle at its junction with the suture and passes the needle to the nurse (Fig. 9-17). The knot can now be formed with an extracorporeal knotting technique.

EXTRACORPOREAL KNOTS

The extracorporeal knot can be tied rapidly and securely. In forming this knot, the "tails" of the suture never enter the abdomen; rather, they are held stationary outside the abdomen. The knot is tied and slid into the abdomen and secured with a knot pusher.

Of the following two techniques, the square knot is preferred to the locking loop knot because it more closely mimics open surgery.

Square knot

1. A single throw (half hitch) or double throw (surgeon's knot) is made with the two ends of the suture. During this time the assistant covers the introducer channel with a finger to prevent loss of the pneumoperitoneum (see Fig. 9-17).

2. *Both ends* of the suture are held by the nondominant hand (Fig. 9-18).
3. The dominant hand now uses a knot pusher to deliver the half hitch into the abdomen (Fig. 9-19). The knot pusher is positioned just beneath the half hitch and is then pushed forward into the 10 mm introducer and downward to the site of the vessel (Fig. 9-20). Both

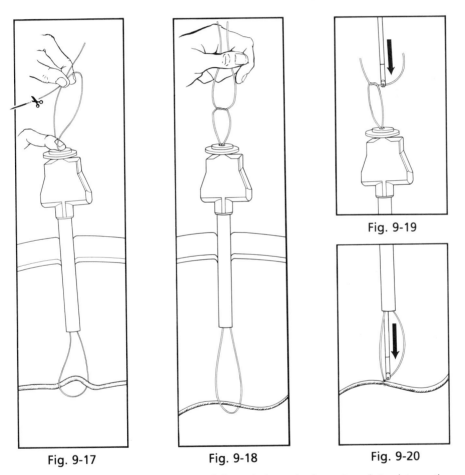

Fig. 9-17   Fig. 9-18   Fig. 9-20

Fig. 9-19

Fig. 9-17 Needle end of suture is delivered through the suture introducer; the needle is cut and the extracorporeal knot can now be formed.

Fig. 9-18 First throw of extracorporeal knot.

Fig. 9-19 Knot pusher placed on suture end. Both ends of the suture are held by the nondominant hand of the surgeon so neither end reenters the trocar.

Fig. 9-20 Knot delivered and tightened around vessel.

ends of the suture remain firmly held by the surgeon's nondominant hand. If a Gazayerli knot pusher is used, as the half hitch is delivered to the surgical site, the jaws of the instrument are opened, thereby firmly cinching the half hitch or surgeon's knot in place.

4. The knot pusher is withdrawn.
5. The assistant again covers the introducer channel with a finger to prevent loss of the pneumoperitoneum.
6. Another half hitch, in the opposite direction, is formed by the surgeon, and steps 2 through 5 are repeated.
7. Additional half hitches in alternating directions are formed and individually delivered, thereby completing the "square knot" or "surgeon's knot."

Locking loop knot

1. Make a single throw (half hitch) with the two suture ends.
2. Hold the knot firmly between thumb and second finger. Designate one end as the "pusher end"; if the integrated suture/knot pusher is being used, the "pusher end" is the end of the suture attached to the plastic pusher.
3. Make three revolutions around the suture strands with the other "free" end of the suture (Fig. 9-21).
4. Insert the free end of the suture *through* the loop beneath the three revolutions (Fig. 9-22).
5. Swing the free end of the suture back and through the loop just below the initial half hitch (see Fig. 9-22).
6. Use a straight clamp to grasp and pull up on the free end of the suture to completely form the knot (Fig. 9-23).
7. Cut the suture tail ¼ inch above the knot.
8. Position the knot pusher above the knot or snap off the end of the integrated suture/knot pusher at the red band to create a plastic knot pusher. Push the shaft of the knot pusher downward while maintaining tension on the "pusher" end of the suture.
9. Use the 5 mm grasper through a different laparoscopic sheath to grasp the sewn tissue in order to relieve any sawing or pulling of the suture on the tissue as the knot is secured.
10. The knot will slide downward as the knot pusher is introduced into the abdomen; the loop of suture beneath the knot will decrease in size.
11. Push the knot until it is securely in place on the tissue. Release tension on the knot and move the pusher back and forth two more times to firmly cinch the knot in place. If the Gazayerli knot pusher

is being used, each time the knot is delivered to the tissue, the jaws of the pusher are opened to further cinch the knot.

12. After securing the knot in place, the hook scissors are introduced through another laparoscopic sheath and the suture is cut ¼ inch from the knot.

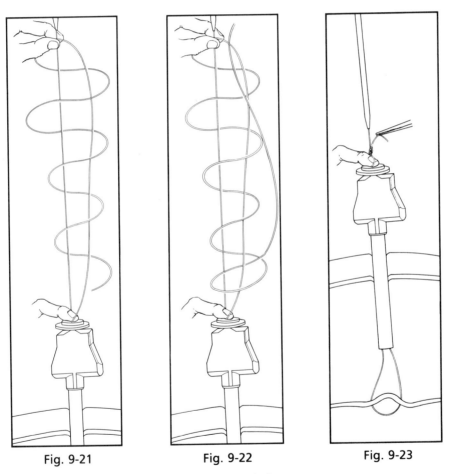

Fig. 9-21   Fig. 9-22   Fig. 9-23

Fig. 9-21 Locking loop knot: initial three revolutions.
Fig. 9-22 Locking loop knot: end of suture is passed around one strand, through the lowest loop, and then through the initial loop.
Fig. 9-23 Locking loop knot: completion of loop knot.

INTRACORPOREAL KNOTS

Intracorporeal knot tying is the most challenging of the suturing and knot-tying techniques. Intracorporeal knotting is used whenever fine sutures are being placed in tissue for reconstruction purposes. It may also be useful to ligate a blood vessel, to approximate tissue planes (e.g., closure of a common bile duct incision or bladder closure), or to create an anastomosis (e.g., ureteroureterostomy). The suture placement is done with either a straight or curved needle; the entire knotting technique is performed within the abdominal cavity. Of the following techniques, the surgeon's knot using a curved needle (the "smiley face" technique) is the most easily learned.

Surgeon's knot—straight needle

Instrumentation A 5 mm needle holder, 10.5 mm reducer cap, 5 mm atraumatic locking grasping forceps (or a second needle holder), 10 mm suture introducer, 5 mm hook scissors, and straight needle attached to only 7 inches of suture (a variety of types are available, including plain gut, chromic, and PDS). Often it is helpful to substitute a second needle holder for the grasping forceps since the suture can also be tightly held in this instrument.

Technique

1. With the 5 mm needle holder, grasp the suture above the junction of the needle and suture so the needle will lie flat against the shaft of the needle holder. Insert the 5 mm needle holder with the needle/suture into the 10 mm suture introducer cannula.
2. After affixing a 10.5 mm reducer cap to the 11 or 12 mm sheath, advance the loaded 10 mm suture introducer through the 11 or 12 mm sheath.
3. Once passed into the abdomen on the 5 mm needle holder, the needle is transferred to a 5 mm grasping forceps that has been passed through another trocar. Position the needle so it lies at a right angle to the needle holder and regrasp the shaft of the needle perpendicularly with the needle holder.
4. Use the 5 mm grasping forceps to depress or hold the targeted tissue taut. Pass the needle through the tissue with the needle holder until the needle tip exits the tissue.
5. Grasp the needle tip with the 5 mm grasping forceps. Draw the suture through the tissue until the remaining tail of suture is about 1 inch in length. It may be helpful to have an assistant hold (i.e., follow) the tail of the suture with a separate grasping forceps,

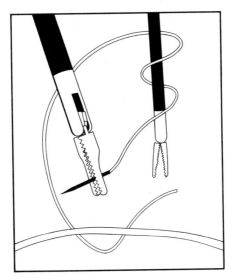

Fig. 9-24 Straight needle: surgeon's knot—formation of initial two loops of the knot.

thereby precluding the surgeon from inadvertently pulling the suture through the tissue. Also the assistant can help deliver the tail of the suture to the surgeon, thereby facilitating the knot-tying process (see step 8).

6. Keep the needle/suture junction oriented toward the now empty needle holder.

7. Wrap two loops of suture around the shaft of the needle holder. This is best accomplished by dipping the tip of the 5 mm needle holder down and around the needle/suture junction; this is done twice (Fig. 9-24). Alternatively, the needle holder can be exchanged for a 5 mm curved grasping forceps; loops of suture can easily be formed around the shaft of the curved grasper by twirling it around the suture.

8. Keeping the needle/suture junction oriented toward the needle holder, grasp the tail of the suture with the needle holder and pull it up through the two newly formed loops. This creates a loose knot (Fig. 9-25).

9. Release and regrasp the tail of the suture nearer the knot; cinch the knot in place by pulling in opposite directions with the needle holder and the 5 mm grasping forceps.

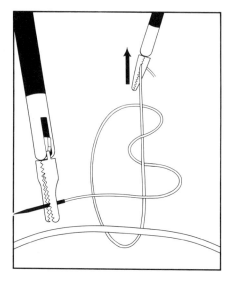

Fig. 9-25 Straight needle: surgeon's knot—cinching the first two loops of the knot.

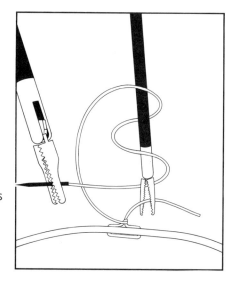

Fig. 9-26 Straight needle: surgeon's knot—creation of second hitch.

10. While holding the needle in the 5 mm grasping forceps, make two additional loops around the needle holder in the *opposite* direction. To do this, circle the 5 mm needle holder down, around, and up the needle/suture junction two times. Grasp the tail of the suture again with the 5 mm needle holder (Fig. 9-26) and pull the tail of the suture through the two newly formed loops to form another hitch (i.e., to "square" the knot). With the grasper, regrasp the

suture nearer the knot and again cinch the knot in place by pulling in the opposite direction, horizontal to the knot, with the needle holder and the 5 mm grasping forceps. Additional half hitches can be placed, depending on the suture material being used (one more hitch for silk suture, two more hitches for chromic suture).

11. Release the needle beside the suture tail. Pick up both strands of the suture with the needle holder.

12. Withdraw the 5 mm grasping forceps and insert the 5 mm hook scissors through a sheath. Holding up on the suture with the needle holder, cut the two suture lines ¼ inch from the knot.

13. Under endoscopic control, the needle and excess suture material are pulled up into the 10 mm suture introducer cannula; remove the needle holder, suture, and suture introducer as a unit from the 11 or 12 mm sheath. Pass the needle to the nurse.

Surgeon's knot—curved needle: "smiley face"

Instrumentation   One 5 mm double-action needle holder and one 5 mm atraumatic locking grasping forceps, 10 mm suture introducer, 10.5 mm reducer cap, 5 mm hook scissors, and curved needle attached to only 7 inches of suture (a variety of types are available, including plain gut, chromic, and PDS). A T-31 needle fits nicely into the 10 mm suture introducer. A second needle holder may be substituted for the grasping forceps.

Technique

1. To insert the curved needle intra-abdominally, place the 5 mm needle holder all the way through the 10 mm suture introducer and grasp the end of the suture. Pull the entire 7-inch length of suture back through the introducer, leaving the needle dangling at the distal end of the introducer. Release the suture from the needle holder and hold the tail of the suture between two fingers.

2. Reinsert the 5 mm needle holder down the length of the introducer and grasp the needle just at the junction of the needle and suture. Keep the needle curve parallel to the needle holder and pull it into the distal end of the introducer.

3. Cut the tail of the suture flush with the introducer.

4. Insert the loaded needle holder and 10 mm introducer through an 11 or 12 mm trocar with a 10.5 mm reducer cap affixed. Advance the needle holder and hence the dangling needle through the introducer into the abdominal cavity.

5. Grasp the needle with 5 mm atraumatic locking grasping forceps passed through another laparoscopic sheath. Open the needle

holder and release the suture. Grasp the needle with the needle holder at the midshaft of the curve in the needle.

6. Grasp or depress the tissue to be sewn with the 5 mm grasping forceps, thereby placing the tissue on tension. Using a rotating wrist motion, drive the needle through the tissue edges. After the tissue is pierced, grasp the tip of the needle with the 5 mm grasping forceps just where the needle tip exits the tissue. Release the needle from the needle holder and regrasp it at its tip. Release the tip of the needle from the grasping forceps. Rotate the needle through the tissue.

7. Use the 5 mm grasping forceps to draw the remaining length of suture into the abdomen. Continue to pull the suture material through the tissue until only a 1-inch tail remains. It may be helpful to have an assistant hold (i.e., follow) the tail of the suture with a separate grasping forceps, thereby precluding the surgeon from inadvertently pulling the suture through the tissue. Also the assistant can help deliver the tail of the suture to the surgeon, thereby facilitating the knot-tying process (see step 11).

8. Reposition the needle in the needle holder so it is being held by the needle holder at the midpoint on the curve of the needle and perpendicular to the field of vision. This makes the needle appear as a "smile" (concave surface directed anterior, convex surface directed posterior).

9. Dip the tip of the grasping forceps around the suture material immediately above its junction with the needle, thereby forming a loop of suture on the shaft of the grasping forceps. (Fig. 9-27, *A*).

10. Pass the tip of the grasping forceps through the curve of the needle between the needle holder and the suture's junction with the needle (Fig. 9-27, *B* and *C*). If a double hitch is desired, make a second loop. Move the loop-carrying grasper closer to the tail of the suture (Fig. 9-27, *D*).

11. Grasp the tail end of the suture with the grasping forceps (Fig. 9-28, *A*).

12. Draw the tail end of the suture through the "formed" suture loop by moving the needle holder and grasping forceps in opposite directions (Fig. 9-28, *B*).

13. Regrasp the tail of the suture material with the grasping forceps closer to the knot and move the two instruments in opposite directions to cinch the knot so it lies flat.

14. Repeat steps 9 through 13, looping the suture material in the opposite direction around the "smiley face" needle to complete the square knot. Additional half hitches can be placed, depending on

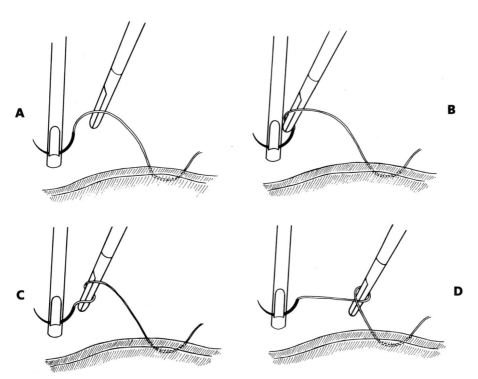

Fig. 9-27 "Smiley face" knot: **A,** Start of initial half hitch; the needle is held in midshaft by the needle holder. The needle is seen face-on in its frontal projection with its convex surface pointed posterior and its concave surface directed anterior (hence it has the appearance of a smile). **B,** Grasper is moved from back surface of suture toward front surface of the needle, around the inside curve of the needle, and then past the back surface of the needle. **C,** This movement allows a loop of suture to form on the shaft of the grasper. If desired, a second loop can be formed on the shaft of the needle holder at this time (i.e., surgeon's knot). **D,** The grasper with its loop of suture is moved closer to the tail end of the suture.

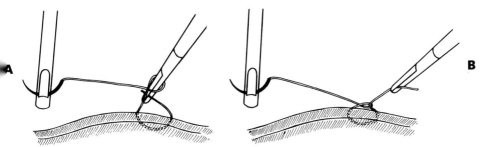

Fig. 9-28 "Smiley face" knot: **A,** Pull the tail of the suture through the loop. **B,** Move the grasper and needle holder away from one another until the first hitch lies flat on the tissue and has been pulled taut.

the suture material being used (one more hitch for silk suture, two more hitches for chromic suture).

15. Release the needle beside the tail of the suture. Pick up both strands of the suture with the needle holder.
16. Withdraw the 5 mm grasping forceps and insert the 5 mm hook scissors through another sheath. While holding up on the suture with the needle holder, cut the sutures ¼ inch from the knot.
17. Under endoscopic control, pull the needle and excess suture material up into the 10 mm suture introducer and then remove the needle holder, suture, and suture introducer as a unit from the 11 or 12 mm laparoscopic sheath.

Triple-twist knot

Instrumentation   A 5 mm needle holder, 5 and 10.5 mm reducer caps, 5 mm atraumatic locking grasping forceps (or a second needle holder), 10 mm suture introducer, 5 mm hook scissors, and *curved* (e.g., T-31) needle attached to 7 inches of suture.

Technique

1. To insert the curved needle intra-abdominally, place the 5 mm needle holder all the way through the 10 mm suture introducer and grasp the end of the suture. Pull the entire length of suture back through the introducer, leaving the needle dangling at the distal end of the introducer. Release the suture from the needle holder and hold the tail of the suture between the two fingers.
2. Reinsert the 5 mm needle holder down the length of the introducer and grasp the needle just at the junction of the needle and suture. Keep the needle curve parallel to the needle holder and pull it into the distal end of the introducer.
3. Cut the suture tail flush with the introducer shaft.
4. Insert the loaded needle holder and 10 mm introducer through an 11 or 12 mm laparoscopic sheath and a 10.5 mm reducer cap attached. Advance the needle holder and hence the needle through the 10 mm introducer into the abdominal cavity.
5. Grasp the needle with 5 mm grasping forceps passed through another laparoscopic sheath. Open the needle holder and release the suture. Grasp the needle with the needle holder at the midshaft of the curve in the needle.
6. Grasp or depress the tissue to be sewn with the 5 mm grasping forceps, thereby placing the tissue on tension. Use a rotating wrist motion to drive the needle through the tissue edges. Grasp the tip of the needle with the 5 mm grasping forceps and steady it. Regrasp

the tip of the needle with the needle holder and rotate the needle through the tissue.

7. If necessary, use the 5 mm grasping forceps to draw the remaining length of suture into the abdomen. Equalize the length of suture strands on either side of the sewn tissue. It may be helpful to have an assistant hold (i.e., follow) the tail of the suture with a separate grasping forceps, thereby precluding the surgeon's inadvertently pulling the suture through the tissue. Also the assistant can help deliver the tail of the suture to the surgeon, thereby facilitating the knot-tying process (see step 11).

8. Grasp the needle with the 5 mm grasping forceps. Open the needle holder and use it to grasp the suture at its juncture with the needle. With the hook scissors, cut the suture so the needle is dangling from the jaws of the needle holder. Now withdraw the needle into the introducer channel and then simultaneously remove the needle holder, needle, and introducer as a unit from the trocar.

9. Reinsert the needle holder through a 5 mm reducer cap placed on the 11 or 12 mm sheath. Grasp one end of the suture so that there is a ½-inch tail (Fig. 9-29). Now rotate the needle holder four times. In this manner three loops of suture are formed around the shaft of the needle holder as it rotates (Fig. 9-30).

10. With the grasping forceps, remove the ½-inch suture tail from the jaws of the needle holder (without dropping any of the loops) (Fig. 9-31).

11. Grasp the opposite free tail of the suture with the needle holder (Fig. 9-32).

12. With the grasping forceps and needle holder each holding a suture tail, begin to move the instruments in opposite directions along a horizontal plane. As the instruments' tips pass each other, dip the grasping forceps downward so it lies below the needle holder, closer to the sewn tissue. This will allow the loops to more easily pass off the needle holder. Continue to pull the instruments in opposite directions. As the loops come off the shaft of the needle holder, a triple throw is formed (Fig. 9-33).

13. The suture is released, and both instruments are moved closer to the knot. Both sides of the suture are grasped closer to the knot, and the two instruments are then moved in opposite directions to further approximate the tissue edges and cinch the knot.

14. A second hitch is completed by repeating steps 9 to 13, forming only two rather than three loops of suture on the needle holder while rotating the needle holder in the *opposite* direction. The loops, when added to the knot, will create a square knot (Fig. 9-34). Ad-

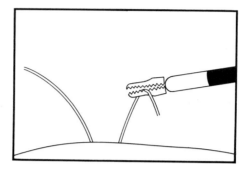

Fig. 9-29 Triple-twist knot: ½-inch tail of suture protrudes from the jaws of the needle holder.

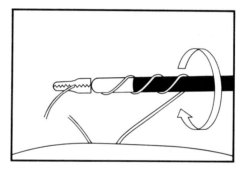

Fig. 9-30 Triple-twist knot: while firmly holding the ½-inch tail of suture, rotate the needle holder four times, thereby creating three loops of suture on the shaft of the needle holder.

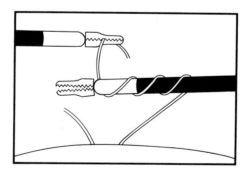

Fig. 9-31 Triple-twist knot: the grasping forceps grasps and removes the ½-inch tail from the jaws of the needle holder.

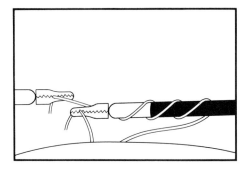

Fig. 9-32 Triple-twist knot: the needle holder grasps the free end of the suture.

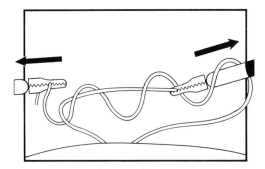

Fig. 9-33 Triple-twist knot: pull the jaws of the needle holder and the jaws of the grasping forceps away from each other. The loops of suture will begin to come off of the shaft of the needle holder. The first hitch of the knot is thus formed and cinched in place.

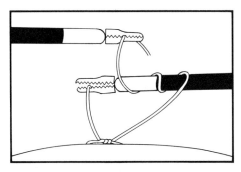

Fig. 9-34 Triple-twist knot: a second hitch (i.e., opposite throw) to "square" the knot is formed by rotating the needle holder in the opposite direction.

ditional half hitches can be placed, depending on the suture material being used (one more hitch for silk suture, two more hitches for chromic suture).

15. Grasp both ends of suture in the needle holder. Withdraw the grasping forceps and insert a hook scissors via another trocar sheath. Cut both strands of suture ¼ inch from the knot and remove the excess suture through the trocar.

360-degree rotational knot

Instrumentation A 5 mm needle holder, 10.5 mm reducer cap, 5 mm atraumatic locking/grasping forceps, 10 mm suture introducer, 5 mm hook scissors, and a curved needle (e.g., T-31) attached to *24 inches* of suture.

Technique

1. To insert the curved needle intra-abdominally, place the 5 mm needle holder all the way through the 10 mm suture introducer and grasp the end of the suture. Pull the entire length of suture back through the introducer, leaving the needle dangling at the distal end of the introducer. Release the suture from the needle holder and hold the tail of the suture between two fingers.

2. Reinsert the 5 mm needle holder down the length of the introducer and grasp the needle just at the junction of needle and suture. Keep the needle curve parallel to the needle holder and pull it into the distal end of the 10 mm suture introducer.

3. Insert the loaded needle holder and 10 mm introducer through an 11 or 12 mm trocar with the 10.5 mm reducer cap affixed.

4. Secure the end of the suture with a clamp so it cannot be inadvertently pulled into the abdomen. Push the needle holder forward until the needle is seen in the abdomen.

5. Grasp the needle with 5 mm grasping forceps passed through another laparoscopic sheath. Open the needle holder and release the suture. Regrasp the needle with the needle holder at the midshaft of the curve in the needle.

6. Grasp or depress the tissue to be sewn with the 5 mm grasping forceps, thereby placing the tissue on tension. Using a rotating wrist motion, drive the needle through the tissue edges. Grasp the tip of the needle with the 5 mm grasping forceps and steady it. Release the needle holder from the needle. Now regrasp the tip of the needle with the needle holder. Release the needle from the grasping forceps. Then rotate the needle through the tissue. The tip of the

grasping forceps can be placed on the tissue just beneath the needle to prevent tearing of the tissue as the needle is delivered through the tissue.

7. Regrasp the needle with the grasping forceps. Reposition the needle holder midway along the curve of the needle. Draw approximately 2 inches of suture through the tissue (Fig. 9-35, A).

8. Hold the tail end of the suture (i.e., portion dangling from the trocar/introducer) so it is taut (i.e., mild tension). Hold the needle end of the suture and needle holder parallel and close to the suture where it exits the needle introducer. There should be no slack in either strand of the suture. The tip of the needle should point at the free strand of the suture; likewise the concave (i.e., inner) curve of the needle should face the free strand of the suture.

9. Rotate the needle holder and needle by turning the needle holder handle 360 degrees three times, thereby creating three twists of suture around the hand-held (free-end) strand of the suture (Fig. 9-35, B).

10. Next, use the needle holder to guide the needle *through* the initial suture loop lying immediately above the sewn tissue; this loop was created by the first twist of the suture (Fig. 9-36, A).

11. Grasp the needle as it exits the initial suture loop with the grasping forceps (Fig. 9-36, A). Transfer the needle back to the needle holder (Fig. 9-36, B). Grasp the hand-held end of the suture with the grasper.

12. Move the needle holder and the grasping forceps in opposite directions, thereby tightening the knot onto the tissue (Fig. 9-36, C). The grasping forceps may need to be repositioned closer to the tissue side of the suture to facilitate tightening the knot.

13. Rotate the needle holder, albeit in the opposite direction, 360 degrees three times (Fig. 9-37). This again results in three twists of the needle-end portion of the suture being formed around the hand-held free strand of the suture.

14. The needle is passed through the loop lying between the first knot and the first loop of the new set of three twists. The needle's tip is grasped by the grasping forceps, and the entire needle is pulled through the loop. The needle can be transferred back to the needle holder. Grasp the suture near the knot (hand-held free-end) with the grasper.

15. The knot is tightened by moving the needle holder and grasping forceps in opposite horizontal directions.

16. Additional alternating throws can be placed, depending on the

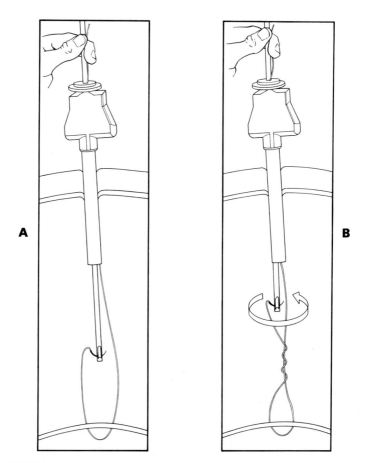

Fig. 9-35 360-degree rotational knot: **A,** Suture passed through tissue. **B,** Needle holder is rotated 360 degrees three times around the free-end side of the strand of suture.

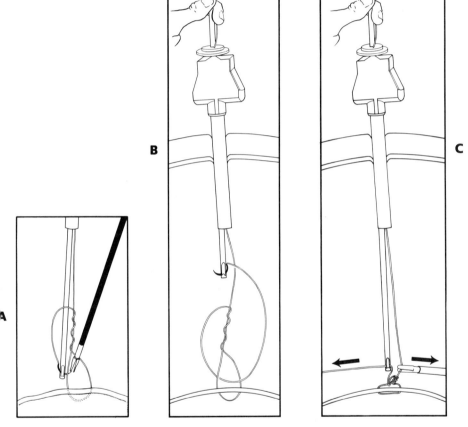

Fig. 9-36 360-degree rotational knot: **A,** Needle tip is passed through the loop closest to the tissue. The tip is then grasped with a grasping forceps and the entire needle is pulled through the loop. **B,** The needle is transferred to the needle holder. **C,** The hand-held strand (i.e., free end) is grasped by the grasping forceps. The needle end of the suture is regrasped by the needle holder. By pulling the grasping forceps and needle holder in opposite directions, the first throw of the knot is formed.

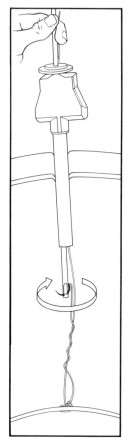

Fig. 9-37 360-degree rotational knot: the needle holder is now rotated 360 degrees three times in the opposite direction to form the second throw of the knot. The steps in Fig. 9-36 are then repeated to cinch the second hitch of the square knot.

suture material used (one more for silk, two more for chromic, and so on).

17. The needle holder is used to grasp both ends of the suture. The grasping forceps are removed, and the hook scissors are inserted. The suture ends are cut ¼ inch from the knot.

18. The remaining suture and needle are withdrawn into the 10 mm suture introducer, and the introducer is removed along with the needle and suture. The needle is given to the nurse.

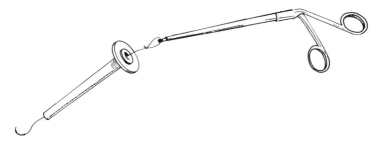

Fig. 9-38 Running suture: seven inches of suture with a terminal slipknot have been backloaded through the 10 mm suture introducer. The slipknot is fed back into the suture introducer.

Running suture

Instrumentation   A 5 mm needle holder, 10.5 mm reducer cap, 5 mm grasping forceps (or a second needle holder), rubber-shod 5 mm grasping forceps, 10 mm suture introducer, 5 mm hook scissors, and straight or curved (e.g., T-31) needle attached to 7 inches of suture. Suture material includes plain gut, chromic, Vicryl, and PDS.

Technique

1. Measure 7 inches of suture and cut the suture at this point.
2. In the end of the suture, make a hangman's knot or slipknot. Tighten the knot around the closed tip of the grasping forceps so that it forms a 5 mm loop. Trim the free tail of the suture so that it barely protrudes from the knot.
3. Pass the 5 mm grasping forceps through the back end of the 10 mm suture introducer and grasp the slipknot of the suture and pull it gently into the suture introducer until the knot is out the back end of the introducer (Fig. 9-38). Now place the knot just inside the introducer. Introduce the needle holder down the length of the introducer and grasp the suture at the junction of the needle and suture (Fig. 9-39). Pull the needle into the distal end of the 10 mm suture introducer.
4. Insert the loaded 10 mm suture introducer through an 11 or 12 mm laparoscopic sheath to which a 10.5 mm reducer cap has been affixed. Advance the needle holder and hence the needle through the introducer into the abdominal cavity.
5. Grasp the needle with 5 mm grasping forceps passed through another laparoscopic sheath. Open the needle holder and release the

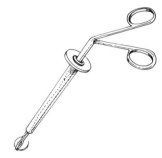

Fig. 9-39 Running suture: the needle holder is advanced through the 10 mm suture introducer; the suture is grasped just where it attaches to the curved needle and retracted into the 10 mm suture introducer.

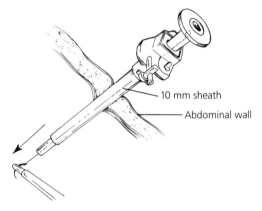

10 mm sheath

Abdominal wall

Fig. 9-40 Running suture: the 10 mm suture introducer is pushed into the 11 or 12 mm trocar. The needle holder is pushed forward and the needle is transferred to the grasping forceps. The needle holder is withdrawn. Needle and entire length of suture with its terminal slipknot are pulled into the abdomen.

suture (Fig. 9-40). Pull the entire length of suture and the slipknot into the abdomen. Grasp the needle with the needle holder at the midshaft of the curve in the needle. Release the grasping forceps from the needle.

6. Grasp or depress the tissue to be sewn with the 5 mm grasping forceps, thereby placing the tissue on tension. Use a rotating wrist motion to drive the needle through the tissue edges. Grasp the tip of the needle with the 5 mm grasping forceps and steady it. Regrasp the tip of the needle with the needle holder and rotate the needle through the tissue.

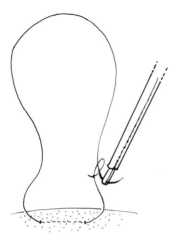

Fig. 9-41 Running suture: after passing the needle through the tissue for the first time, the needle is passed through the loop of the slipknot. The needle is grasped by the grasping forceps and completely pulled through the slipknot, thereby securing the first knot of the running suture.

7. Pull the suture through the tissue with the needle holder until the slipknot abuts the sewn tissue. Now pass the needle through the loop of the slipknot (Fig. 9-41). Grasp the tip of the needle with the grasping forceps and pull the entire needle through the loop of the slipknot. Continue to pull on the needle until the suture is pulled completely through the loop. The slipknot should now be tightly cinched on the sewn tissue, thereby completing the first knot of the running suture.

8. Regrasp the needle with the needle holder and continue the running suture through the tissues by repeating step 6. After the needle is rotated through the tissue with the needle holder, then the grasping forceps are used to grasp the needle. The needle holder is then freed from the tip of the needle and used to regrasp the needle at the midpoint of its curve so another pass through the tissue can be taken. The rubber-shod grasper can be used by the assistant to "follow" the suture and pull it taut with each pass through the tissue.

9. When the last bite of tissue is taken with the suture, leave the loop of suture loose.

10. Now reposition the needle in the needle holder so it is being held at the midpoint on the curve of the needle ("smiley face") and that

the concave surface of the needle is directed anteriorly (see discussion of the "smiley face" knot).

11. Dip the tip of the grasping forceps around the backside of the suture material directly extending from the needle.

12. Pass the tip of the grasping forceps through the curve of the needle between the needle holder and the suture end of the needle, thereby forming a loop of suture on the shaft of the grasping forceps. Repeat this motion.

13. Grasp the loose last loop of suture at its midpoint with the grasping forceps.

14. Draw the midpoint of the loose loop through the suture loops on the grasping forceps by moving the needle holder and grasping forceps in opposite directions, thereby moving the suture loops from off the shaft and tip of the grasping forceps.

15. Regrasp the suture on the needle side, closer to the knot, with the needle holder. Again, move the instruments in opposite horizontal directions to cinch the first throw.

16. Repeat steps 10 through 15, but loop the suture material in the opposite direction around the needle to complete the square knot. Add an additional throw for silk suture or form two separate, additional throws for chromic suture.

17. Release the needle alongside the knot. Pick up the three strands of suture with the needle holder.

18. Withdraw the 5 mm grasping forceps and insert the 5 mm hook scissors through a 5 mm laparoscopic sheath. While holding up on the three strands with the needle holder, cut the sutures ¼ inch from the knot.

19. Pull the needle and excess suture material up into the 10 mm suture introducer cannula and then remove the needle holder, suture, and 10 mm suture introducer as a unit from the 11 or 12 mm trocar. Pass the needle to the nurse.

SUMMARY

After mastering the basic suturing and knot-tying techniques, the surgeon can be considered to possess complete laparoscopic capability. It may require concentrated practice to become facile with all of these knots, but the reward is the confidence to undertake any laparoscopic surgical procedure that may arise. In most instances the mechanical devices used to achieve hemostasis and approximation of tissues, such as clips and staples, will provide a quicker and more efficient method of achieving these tasks. However, the ability to suture and tie laparoscopic knots may on occasion be the only way to complete a laparoscopic procedure and avert converting the procedure to a laparotomy. It is also the essential first step for learning to perform a variety of laparoscopic reconstructive procedures.

■ ■ ■

We would like to thank Drs. E.J. Reddick and H. Toppel for their excellent work in teaching laparoscopic suturing.

REFERENCES
1. Soper NJ, Hunter JG. Suturing and knot tying in laparoscopy. Surg Clin North Am 72:1139-1152, 1992.
2. Ko S, Airan MC. Therapeutic laparoscopic suturing techniques. Surg Endoscopy 6:41, 1992.

CHAPTER 10

Laparoscopic Clips and Staples

Elspeth M. McDougall, Ralph V. Clayman, and Nathaniel J. Soper

Surgical clips and staples have been adapted for use through the laparoscope. Laparoscopic titanium clips and staples can be used to secure and ligate vessels, close luminal/pelvic abdominal structures such as the ureter, bladder, or bowel, and to reapproximate tissue edges. The clips and staples provide a more rapid means for completing these tasks than standard laparoscopic suturing techniques. In this chapter the various types of clips and staples are reviewed and the techniques for applying them are described.

INSTRUMENTS

Clips

Clips are available in two forms: occlusive (i.e., clothespin type) and tacking. The *occlusive* clips come in lengths of 6, 9, and 11 mm and are excellent for occluding a vessel (Table 10-1). The occlusive clip applier

Table 10-1   Occlusive clips

Clip	Producer*	Clip length (inner) (mm)	No. of staples	Handle longevity†	Trocar sheath size	Features
EL214	E	5.2	1	ND	10	1
EL314	E	8.8	1	ND	10	1
EL414	E	12.5	1	ND	10	1
EM320	E	8.4	20	D	10	1,2
ER320	E	8.4	20	D	10	1,2
EndoClip M	A	6.0	20	D	10	1
EndoClip ML	A	9.0	20	D	10	1
EndoClip L	A	11.0	15	D	10	1
EndoClip Palm M	A	6.0	15	D	10	1
EndoClip Palm ML	A	9.0	15	D	10	1
EndoClip Palm L	A	11.0	15	D	10	1

Features

1 = Rotating head feature allows the shaft and tip of the instrument to be rotated without moving the handles of the instrument.

2 = Automatic loading.

*E = Ethicon; A = Autosuture (U.S. Surgical Corp.).

†ND = nondisposable; D = disposable.

is passed into the abdomen via a ≥10 mm port. The tips of the clip are approximated by the jaws of the clip applier before the closure of the body of the clip (Fig. 10-1).

The *tacking* clips close in either a rectangular or B configuration (Fig. 10-2) (Table 10-2). These clips are used to tack Marlex mesh to the

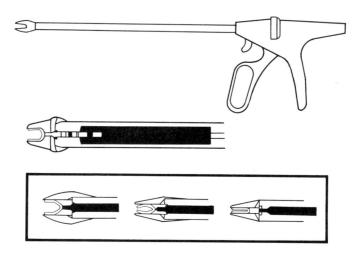

Fig. 10-1 Disposable multiload occlusive clip applier: detail of firing mechanism and clip closure.

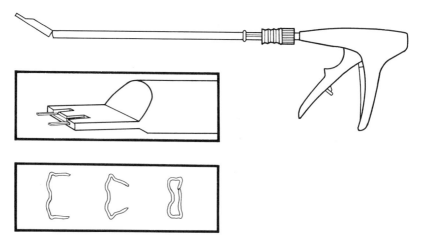

Fig. 10-2 Disposable surgical tacking stapler: detail of firing mechanism and clip closure.

Table 10-2   Tacking clips and staplers

Tacking clips	Producer*	Outer clip dimension (L × W) (mm)	Inner clip dimension (L × W) (mm)	No. of staples	Handle longevity†	Trocar sheath size	Features
EAS 60	E	4.4 × 3.6	3.2 × 2.6	25	D	11	1, 3 (60 degrees), Rectangular closure
EMS 30	E	5.3 × 3.7	4.2 × 2.6	30	D	11	1, 2, Rectangular closure
E 9	E			1	ND	11	1, Rectangular closure
Endohernia	A	4.8 × 5.8	3.0 × 4.8	10	D	12	2, 3 (40 degrees), 4, "B" closure

Staplers	Producer*	Staple line length (mm)	Staple rows	Staple sizes‡	Handle longevity†	Port size (mm)	Features
EndoGIA 30	A	30	6	2.5	D	12	1, 4
EndoGIA 60	A	60	6	3.8	D	15	1, 4, 5
EndoTA 60	A	60	3	4.8	D	15	1, 4
Endopath 30	E	30	6	3.85	D	12	1, 4
Endopath 60	E	60	4	4.5	D	18	1, 4

Features
1 = Rotating head feature allows the shaft and tip of the instrument to be rotated without moving the handles of the instrument.
2 = Automatic loading.
3 = The jaws of the clip applier can be articulated.
4 = Additional staple cartridges can be loaded into same disposable handle.
5 = Pneumatic firing.
*E = Ethicon; A = Autosuture (U.S. Surgical Corp.).
†ND = nondisposable; D = disposable.
‡EndoGIA 30 and 60 are both available in 2.5, 3.8, and 4.8 sizes; Endopath 30 and 60 are both available in 3.85 and 4.5 sizes.

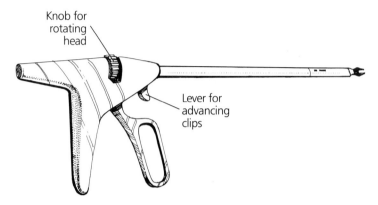

Fig. 10-3 Disposable multiload clip applier.

abdominal sidewall during a hernia repair or to close incisions in the peritoneum (e.g., ureterolysis). The tacking clip applier is passed into the abdomen via a ≥11 mm port.

In general the clip appliers have a ≥10 mm shaft. They may be either a multiload disposable type or a single-load reusable type. The latter can be used repeatedly; however, after each clip application, the clip applier must be removed from the abdomen and reloaded. Despite this drawback the advantage of the reusable clip applier is the cost savings. After making the initial investment in the clip applier (approximately six times the cost of a disposable unit), one has to purchase only a rack of clips for each case.

The multiload disposable clip applier comes with 15 to 30 clips already loaded in the applier (Fig. 10-3). These instruments have a shaft that can be rotated to help align the tip of the clip applier with the structure to be occluded or tacked. Also, this clip applier is capable of firing clips in rapid succession; as such, it can greatly facilitate a laparoscopic procedure in which multiple vascular structures need to be secured and cut (e.g., bowel resection or nephrectomy) or when the peritoneum needs to be resurfaced.

Staples

All appliers of laparoscopic staples are currently available only in a disposable form (Fig. 10-4). The staple sizes range from 2.5 to 4.8 mm; the length of each row of staples is 3 or 6 cm; usually each staple cartridge delivers six separate rows of staples. As the staples are pushed into the tissue and closed, a knife cuts the tissue between staple lines

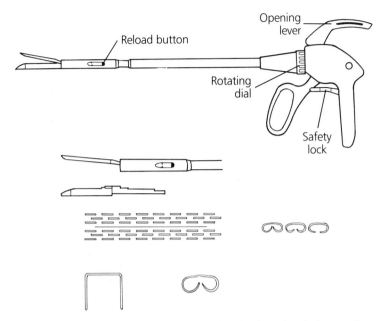

Fig. 10-4 Disposable surgical stapler. This stapler can be reloaded up to four times, if necessary, during the same procedure; it provides for six rows of staples and incises the tissue between rows 3 and 4.

Fig. 10-5 Nondisposable single-load clip applier.

3 and 4 (Table 10-2). The smaller staples are used to occlude vascular structures, whereas the larger staples are used to secure bulkier tissues (e.g., the bowel wall, a vaginal cuff, or a bladder cuff).

LOADING AND FIRING CLIPS
Single load

The reusable clip appliers are hand loaded, one clip at a time (Fig. 10-5). Some models also have a shaft that can be rotated to aid in clip alignment. The *single-load clips* are kept in a rack, and the empty jaws of the clip applier are advanced over a clip until a click is felt; the clip should then rest snugly within the jaws of the clip applier. The loaded clip applier is withdrawn from the rack of clips. The clip is applied by slowly squeezing the handles of the clip applier together. It is important when introducing the loaded instrument into the 10 mm trocar sheath that no force be applied to the handles of the clip applier lest the clip be partly closed and thus fall from the jaws of the clip applier. Accordingly, it is helpful to hold on to just the back handle of the loaded reusable clip applier until it has been maneuvered to the surgical site; then both the front and back handles can be held in the surgeon's grasp.

Multiload

With the disposable clip appliers, a rack of 15 to 30 clips is preloaded. The instrument is held like a gun, with the index finger on the trigger of the clip applier (U.S. Surgical Corp.). By pulling the trigger mechanism, a clip is loaded into the jaws of the clip applier. The handles can then be squeezed together to deliver the clip onto the tissue. The handles cannot be squeezed together unless the trigger has been pulled first and a clip loaded; however, if the clip happens to fall out of the jaws of the clip applier, the handles can still be squeezed together and the jaws apposed. Accordingly, before squeezing the handles together, the surgeon must first check the jaws of the clip applier to "see" that a clip is present.

Also, if the trigger and the handles of the clip applier are simultaneously squeezed, the loading mechanism may become jammed and a new clip applier will be needed. To prevent this from happening, when maneuvering the clip applier, the index finger should be kept off the trigger; only when a clip is to be loaded should the index finger be moved to the trigger. At this point the bottom three digits holding the front handle of the clip applier are moved so that the clip applier is held only by its back handle, thereby precluding any possibility of simultaneously squeezing the handles together while the clip is being loaded. Once the clip is loaded, the index finger is again moved away from the trigger and the bottom three fingers are moved forward so that they hold the front handle of the clip applier while the back handle is cradled against the thenar/hypothenar eminence of the surgeon's hand. The front handle can now be squeezed toward the back handle at the surgeon's discretion, thereby closing the clip.

Another type of disposable multiload clip applier is self-loading (Ethicon Endosurgery). There is no loading trigger. Again, with this instrument it is important to hold only the back handle while maneuvering the instrument and to grasp both handles only when ready to secure the tissue with a clip. After a clip is squeezed onto the surgical site, the handles are released. As the front handle moves forward, the jaws of the clip applier open and another clip is automatically spring-fed into its jaws (see Table 10-1).

LOADING AND FIRING STAPLES

The staple appliers are assembled so that the jaws are closed when the device is inserted through the ≥12 mm sheath. A lever located on the top of the device or on the handle is raised from the body of the applier, thereby opening the jaws that hold the two parts of the staple cartridge. This lever is used to close and lock the jaws of the stapler on the tissue that is to be approximated and cut. Also, there is usually a *safety lock* between the handles of the applier; this prevents the handles from being inadvertently squeezed together, which would fire the staples prematurely. The lock between the handles must be swung downward to allow the handles to be apposed. Squeezing the handles of the applier together simultaneously discharges all six rows of staples and cuts the tissue. The handles can then be allowed to return to their more separated "resting" position. Next, by releasing the lever on the body of the applier, the jaws of the stapler are opened so that the applier can be withdrawn from the stapled and incised tissue.

Some staple appliers can be reloaded with a fresh cartridge of staples. To do this, the reloading button is pushed and the spent cartridge is removed. A fresh staple cartridge is then inserted onto the staple jaw, which lies opposite the anvil jaw of the applier.

METHOD OF APPLICATION
Clips: occlusive

Vascular occlusion
1. The vessel to be occluded is dissected circumferentially from the surrounding fat and connective tissue. A 360-degree "window" must be created around the vessel. The vessel is stripped until its adventitial surface is clearly visible; curved grasping forceps and electrosurgical scissors or a right-angled, hook-type electrosurgical probe are most helpful to accomplish this task.
2. When finished, the curved grasping forceps can be inserted behind the vessel so that the tips are easily visualized emerging on the other side of the vessel. The "window" should be extended 1.5 to 2.0 cm along the vessel.
3. The clip applier is inserted through a ≥10 mm trocar, which enters the surgical field *perpendicular* to the sidewall of the vessel. Also, the clip applier should enter the field of view at an oblique-to-perpen-

dicular angle to the laparoscope. This enables the surgeon to view the clip applier side-on instead of end-on as it approaches the vessel.

4. With the *nondisposable* clip applier, the clip rests in the jaws of the clip applier from the moment the applier is passed into the 10 mm port. Care must be taken not to dislodge the clip from the clip applier while passing the applier to the surgical site; also, the handles of the clip applier must not be inadvertently squeezed during passage of the clip applier; if this occurs, the clip may fall from the jaws of the applier. With the *disposable* multiload clip applier, the clip applier is not loaded until the clip applier is near the vessel.

   Before passing the "loaded" clip applier over the vessel, the surgeon should rotate the shaft of the clip applier so that he or she can "see" that there is definitely a clip within the jaws of the clip applier. If this is not done and the clip has indeed fallen out of the jaws of the clip applier, the "empty" jaws of the clip applier may inadvertently be applied to the vessel; the sharp edges of the applier's "empty" jaws can cut the vessel, and significant hemorrhage ensue.

5. Closed grasping forceps are passed alongside the vessel wall farthest from the clip applier (i.e., far wall). As the grasping forceps push the vessel wall toward the clip applier, the jaws of the clip applier are placed across the vessel. This allows the jaws of the clip applier to pass completely over the vessel. Both tips of the clip applier's jaws should be easily visible beyond the far wall of the vessel (Fig. 10-6, *A*).

6. The handles of the applier are slowly squeezed to the half-closed position. The ends of the clip come together. The partially closed clip assumes a teardrop shape as it encompasses the full circumference of the vessel. At this moment the clip can be *slid* up or down along the vessel (Fig. 10-6, *A*). This maneuver enables the surgeon to place the clips in such a manner that the longest possible length of vessel is exposed, thereby allowing the surgeon to place additional clips on the vessel and still have ample room to incise it.

7. Once in the correct position, the handles of the applier are squeezed firmly together; the clip is compressed and flattened onto the sides of the vessel wall, thereby occluding the vessel. The ends of the clip should touch each other with no intervening tissue (Fig. 10-6, *B*). The grip on the handles is relaxed; the jaws open and the clip applier is withdrawn straightaway from the vessel (Fig. 10-6, *C*).

8. This procedure is repeated until, for a large vessel (e.g., splenic or renal artery or vein), there are three clips on the proximal side of the blood vessel and two clips on the distal side of the vessel (Fig. 10-7).

9. The clip applier is removed. Through the same ≥10 mm trocar (now covered with a 5.5 mm reducer), 5 mm laparoscopic scissors are

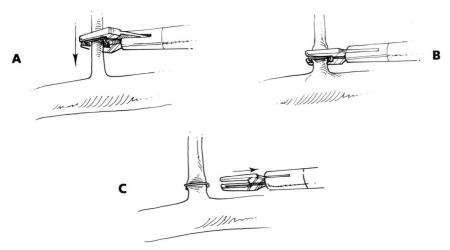

Fig. 10-6 Application of occlusive clips. **A,** Clip completely around vessel. The handles of the clip applier are squeezed just enough to cause the tip of the clip applier to close around the vessel; the clip now forms a metal ring around the vessel, and in this configuration it can be moved farther down on the vessel. **B,** The handles of the clip applier are squeezed firmly together, thereby closing the clip on the vessel. **C,** The surgeon's grip on the handles of the clip applier is relaxed, allowing the jaws of the clip applier to open so it can be removed from the vessel. The clip traverses the entire diameter of the vessel and remains firmly attached to the vessel.

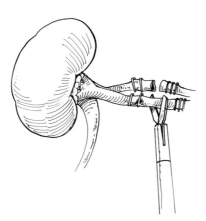

Fig. 10-7 Five clips have been applied (in this case) to the renal artery and then to the renal vein. The artery was cut first; now the vein is being cut. Note that three clips remain on the arterial stump and will likewise remain on the venous stump.

inserted and the vessel is transected between clips two and three so these clips remain on the stump of the vessel (see Fig. 10-7).

Clips: tacking

Resurfacing the peritoneal cavity

1. A pair of 5 mm atraumatic grasping forceps are introduced, one via a lateral 5 mm port and the other via a medial 5 mm port. The first grasper holds the incised lateral edge of the peritoneum, and the second grasper holds the opposite incised medial edge of the peritoneum. The two edges are held together by placing the grasping forceps "tip-to-tip," similar to the manner in which the skin is held upward and apposed with two fine forceps before placing a skin clip (Fig. 10-8).

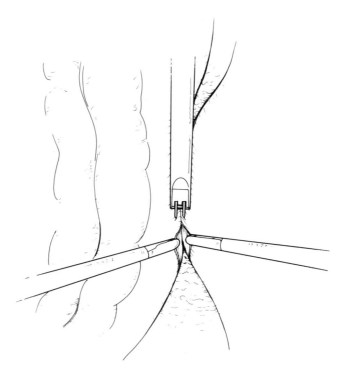

Fig. 10-8 Resurfacing the peritoneal cavity using tacking clips to close the peritoneotomy. To place the initial clip, the two cut edges of the peritoneum are approximated with two grasping forceps. The clip is applied just where the peritoneal edges touch one another.

Alternatively, the lateral and medial atraumatic graspers are positioned on the medial and lateral edges of the peritoneum respectively 2 to 3 cm away from one another. The lateral grasper is then used to pull the medial edge of the peritoneum 1.0 to 1.5 cm over the lateral edge of the peritoneum; the medial grasper is used to pull the lateral edge of the peritoneum 1.0 to 1.5 cm over the medial edge of the peritoneum. As such, the tip of the lateral grasper lies lateral to the tip of the medial grasper; accordingly, the medial and lateral edges of the peritoneum lying between the two grasping forceps are thus made to cross over one another, thereby forming an X at the point where the two edges of the peritoneum cross (Fig. 10-9).

2. The tacking clip applier is inserted through a ≥11 mm laparoscopic

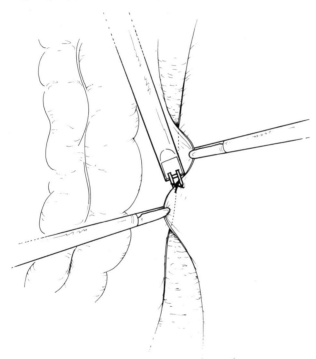

Fig. 10-9 Resurfacing the peritoneal cavity. Two graspers are placed on the cut peritoneal edge. The medial edge of the peritoneum is moved laterally until it overlies the lateral edge of the peritoneum. Where the two edges cross (X), a tacking clip will be placed.

sheath so that it enters the surgical field perpendicular to the grasped edge of the peritoneum and at an oblique or right angle to the laparoscope.

3. When the tip of the disposable clip applier lies just above the peritoneum, a clip is loaded. If a reusable clip applier is being used, the tacking clip should have been loaded before passing the clip applier into the abdomen.
4. The jaws of the clip applier are pushed against the peritoneum, visibly indenting it either just beneath the two graspers ("tip-to-tip" arrangement) or between the graspers (X arrangement). (The latter method was described by Nelson Stone, M.D., Mount Sinai School of Medicine, New York.)
5. The handles of the clip applier are squeezed slowly and firmly together.
6. As the clip is fired into the peritoneum, the ends of the legs of the clip can be seen as they initially exit the jaws in a straight fashion parallel to each other. At this point the clip's body should straddle the cut edges of the peritoneum and the tips of the clip should lie on either side of the peritoneum. Now the handles of the clip applier are squeezed together; the ends of the clip begin to square or curl inward toward one another, thereby simultaneously piercing the medial and lateral edges of the peritoneum. The handles are further apposed until the clip assumes a rectangular or B configuration.
7. The surgeon's grip on the handles is relaxed; the jaws open. If it is reusable, the clip applier is withdrawn from the abdomen and reloaded; if the applier is a multiload disposable type, it is reloaded at the surgical site.
8. After placing the first clip, the two approximated (i.e., clipped) edges of the peritoneum can be grasped with one pair of forceps and held. The tip-to-tip or X arrangement is no longer needed. The clip applier is positioned so it again straddles the cut edges of peritoneum just beneath the grasping forceps. Another clip is applied (Fig. 10-10). This process is continued until the peritoneum has been completely resurfaced.

Staples: tissue

Securing the bowel

1. When performing bowel surgery with the use of stapling devices, one must carefully plan trocar placement. Usually the primary prob-

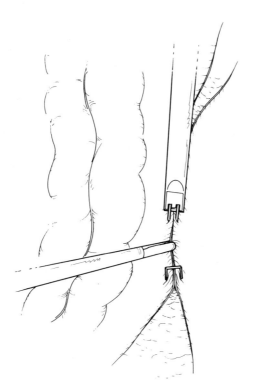

Fig. 10-10 Resurfacing the peritoneal cavity. After placing the initial clip, both edges of the peritoneum are grasped with one grasping forceps. Subsequent clips are placed as the forceps and clip applier are walked down the cut edges of the peritoneum.

lem is "getting far enough away" from the operative site with the trocars, since the staplers must be inserted completely into the 12 mm sheaths before the jaws are opened. Also, when 60 mm linear stapling devices are being used, these must be inserted through larger trocars, either 15 mm (U.S. Surgical Corp.) or 18 mm (Ethicon Endosurgery).

2. The peritoneum overlying the root of the mesentery of the bowel to be resected is scored, either with an electrosurgical scissors or with a hook-tipped electrosurgical probe. Similar to open surgery, the peritoneum is incised up to the bowel wall at each extremity of the planned resection. The mesentery is then divided, with hemostasis

achieved using the occlusive clips (Fig. 10-11) or a 30 mm EndoGIA vascular load (U.S. Surgical Corp.).

3. The stapling device, with the jaws closed, is inserted through a >12 mm trocar. The device should enter the surgical field perpendicular to the axis of the bowel to be divided. Also, the stapling device should enter the surgical field oblique or perpendicular to the laparoscope so that the jaws of the stapling device can easily be viewed side-on (obliquely) rather than coaxially.

4. The lever on the upper body or handle of the stapling device is released; the jaws of the device are thus opened maximally and are placed across the bowel just at the site where the mesentery has been scored on the bowel wall itself. The tips of the stapler's jaw must extend beyond the far wall of the bowel. The lever on the stapling device is then returned to its locked position, thereby closing the jaws on the bowel. The surgeon must carefully examine the end of the stapling device to observe the "cut" line. All tissue to be stapled and incised must lie proximal to the cut line. The stapling device is rotated until the undersurface of the stapling device can be clearly seen; all of the bowel tissue to be cut must again lie proximal to the

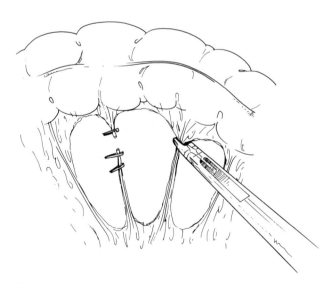

Fig. 10-11 Clip applier is used to secure the mesenteric vessels, which are then divided.

cut line on the *reverse* side of the stapling device; the mesentery should not be included in the line of division. The stapling device is then rotated back to its original position.

5. The horizontal intervening span of plastic between the two handles on the stapler is now swung downward. The handles are firmly squeezed together, delivering all six rows of staples and incising the tissue between rows 3 and 4.

6. Pressure on the handles is relaxed. The lever on the stapler is raised and the jaws of the stapling device are opened. The stapling device is withdrawn from the bowel.

7. The lever is returned to its locked position, thus closing the empty jaws of the stapling device so it can be removed from its laparoscopic port.

8. The staple line is inspected for any bleeding. The extremities of the staple line are examined carefully to ensure that the entire width of the bowel has been controlled with the staples themselves.

9. The other end of the bowel specimen is secured and divided in a similar manner with a second firing of the stapler (Fig. 10-12). The surgeon then proceeds either with an intracorporeal or extracorpo-

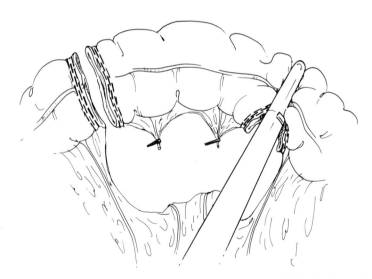

Fig. 10-12 The 30 mm GIA stapler is used to ligate and divide both ends of the selected bowel segment.

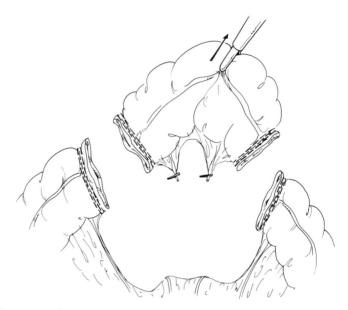

Fig. 10-13 The resected segment is removed from the operative field.

real anastomosis and removes the isolated tissue either by extending the incision or placing the resected specimen in a nylon entrapment sack before its removal (Fig. 10-13) (see Chapter 8).

Removal of the pelvic adnexa

The tube and ovary may be removed using a method similar to that described for securing a bladder cuff:

1. The pelvic adnexa are dissected free from any abnormal attachments such as adhesions to the bowel. The planned pedicle must be clearly isolated from surrounding structures with clear identification of the ureter.
2. A 5 mm traumatic grasping forceps placed through a contralateral sheath is used to elevate and properly expose the adnexa.
3. A sizing device is placed through a 12 mm ipsilateral sheath. The device should enter in an orientation perpendicular to the laparoscope and in proper alignment for placement of the staple line (Fig. 10-14, *A*). The thickness of the pedicle is assessed by this device, which determines the size of the staple.
4. The sizing device is replaced by the stapling device. The stapler is aligned exactly the same as the sizing device and placed over the

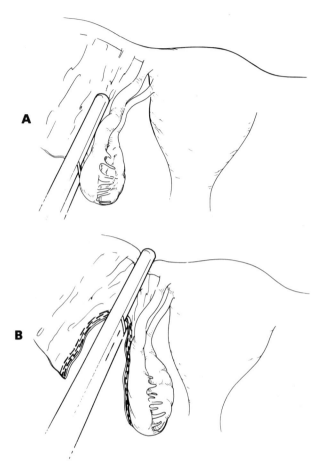

Fig. 10-14 A, The stapling device is carefully positioned on the pedicle and inspected prior to placement of the staples. **B,** The remaining portion of the pedicle may be stapled and excised as needed.

pedicle to be cut. This placement requires very careful inspection of both sides of the staple line as described above. Since the tip will not protrude beyond the tissue to be cut, one must pay close attention to the location of the "cut" line.
5. The "safety" is then released, staples applied, stapler released, and removed from the incision and from the patient as described above. The staple line is carefully inspected.
6. The above procedures are repeated for subsequent pedicles, as needed (Fig. 10-14, *B*).

Staples: vascular

This method is the same as that for applying the tissue staples. However, a major artery and vein such as the renal pedicle should not be occluded en masse with a single firing of the vascular stapler. If this is to be used for securing a broad vein, then the artery should be cleanly dissected from the vein and secured separately with 5 clips, as previously described. The vein is cleared of surrounding tissue, and the stapler is applied following the previously described steps and precautions.

TROUBLESHOOTING

Problem: Cannot load a clip (NB: Semiautomatic clip applier).
Solution:
1. Squeeze the handles together; the previous clip may have fallen out of the jaws of the clip applier. A new clip cannot be loaded until the handles have been squeezed together and released.
2. Be certain you are not exerting any pressure on the handles of the clip applier. Hold the clip applier by the back handle only while loading a clip.
3. Be certain you are not putting undue torque on the shaft of the clip applier. If the shaft is bent even slightly, the clips will not load properly.

Problem: Cannot get all of the tissue proximal to the "cut" line of the tissue stapler.
Solution: Via a 5 mm port, use a curved grasper to hook the far margin of the tissue to be secured. Now the tissue can be pulled into the jaws of the stapling device. Close the jaws when the tissue is well proximal to the "cut" line.

Problem: Not all tissue within the jaws of the stapler has been cut.
Solution: The stapler was not properly placed on the tissue. Either a complete window around the far margin of the tissue was not developed, or the stapling device was fired before the surgeon made certain that the tissue to be stapled lay proximal to the cut line on *both* the front and back sides of the stapler. Use a second staple cartridge to secure and incise the remaining tissue.

REFERENCES

1. Kerbl K, Chandhoke P, McDougall E, Figenshau RS, Stone AM, Clayman RV. Laparoscopic *stapled* bladder closure: Laboratory and clinical experience. J Urol 149:1437-1441, 1993.
2. Kerbl K, Clayman RV, Chandhoke PS, McDougall E, Stone AM, Figenshau RS. Ligation of the renal pedicle during laparoscopic nephrectomy: Staples versus clips. J Laparoendoscopic Surgery 3:9-12, 1993.
3. Chandhoke PS, Clayman RV, Kerbl K, Figenshau RS, McDougall EM, Kavoussi LR, Stone AM. Laparoscopic ureterectomy: Initial clinical experience. J Urol 149:992-998, 1993.
4. Soper NJ, Brunt LM, Fleshman J Jr, Dunnegan DL, Clayman RV. Laparoscopic small bowel resection and anastomosis. Surg Laparosc Endosc 3:6-12, 1993.

CHAPTER 11

Exiting the Abdomen

Howard N. Winfield and Ralph V. Clayman

Inspection
Irrigation
Sheath Removal
Pain Control
Troubleshooting

INSPECTION

On completion of the specific laparoscopic procedure, a survey of the surgical field is performed to look for bleeding or other visceral injuries. The intra-abdominal pressure is lowered to ≤5 mm Hg; this will allow any venotomy previously tamponaded by the 15 mm Hg pneumoperitoneum to be recognized. Next, the peritoneal cavity is scanned from the pelvic region to the upper abdominal quadrants to rule out any previously unrecognized injury to the abdominal viscera.

IRRIGATION

At this point 500 to 2000 cc of irrigation solution may be introduced into the abdominal cavity. The irrigant may contain 500 mg of cefazolin (Ancef) in the first liter; *no* heparin is used in this irrigant. As the irrigant is filling the abdomen, the surgeon can further examine the abdomen for any site of bleeding and for any yellow or brown discoloration of the fluid. The latter is a sign of an unrecognized bowel injury.

Whether to aspirate the irrigant or leave it in place is a controversial subject. Some surgeons prefer to aspirate the fluid, whereas others leave the fluid in place, believing that it may decrease adherence of the bowel

to the laparoscopic port sites and lessen the chances of any postlapa-
roscopic adhesions or infection (i.e., pelvic abscess or peritonitis). Definitive proof in support of the latter hypothesis is lacking. However,
if irrigant fluid is left in place in the male patient, particularly if a hernia
repair or pelvic lymph node dissection has been done, significant and
at times massive hydroceles may acutely develop in the early postoperative period when the patient begins to ambulate. This fluid is slowly
resorbed over a 7- to 10-day period, resulting in resolution of the hydroceles.

SHEATH REMOVAL

The final step in the laparoscopic procedure is to remove the laparoscopic sheaths. The 10 mm laparoscope is used to examine the point
of entry of each of the secondary sheaths into the abdomen. There
should be no bleeding from these sites. Next, a 5 mm laparoscope may
be introduced into one of the 5 mm secondary sheaths, and the site of
entry of the initial ≥10 mm sheath into the abdomen is again carefully
examined for any bleeding from the peritoneal side of the entry site
(Fig. 11-1).

The primary ≥10 mm sheath is removed from the abdominal cavity.
The assistant places a finger over the skin incision so that the pneu-

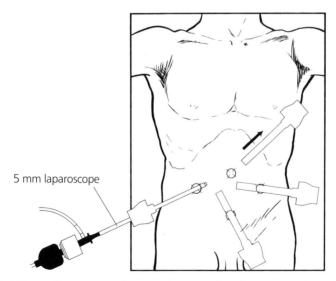

5 mm laparoscope

Fig. 11-1 A 5 mm laparoscope is passed to examine the entry points of the ≥10
mm sheaths and to monitor the fascial closure of the ≥10 mm trocar sites.

moperitoneum can be maintained. A visual inspection is done with the laparoscope to see whether there is bleeding from the area of the peritoneotomy.

Next, the incision through the fascia and subcutaneous tissues, which was made for the ≥10 mm trocar, is closed with 0 and 4-0 absorbable sutures, respectively. The former is done using a horseshoe-shaped needle (TT-3). An S-curved retractor or Sinn retractor is used to retract the skin and expose the fascia. The fascia on either side of the incision is grasped with a Kocher or an Allis clamp (Fig. 11-2, *A*). A single figure-of-eight suture is placed in the fascia (Fig. 11-2, *B*) This is usually

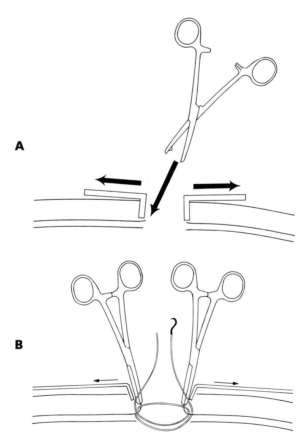

Fig. 11-2 A, Sinn retractors used to expose fascia. **B,** Kocher clamps are affixed to the fascia to facilitate suture placement.

sufficient to close the fascial defect completely. The pneumoperitoneum is maintained during placement of the suture. *This part of the procedure is done under direct endoscopic control via the 5 mm laparoscope placed through one of the secondary sheaths.* As such, the fascial suture is monitored as it is placed to guarantee that no bowel segments are entrapped by the stitch.

If a secondary ≥10 mm trocar was placed during the procedure, this sheath is removed next. The removal of this sheath and the closure of the port site are identical to the procedure just described for removing the initial ≥10 mm trocar.

After all ≥10 mm sheaths have been removed and the fascia closed, all but the laparoscope-bearing 5 mm sheaths are pulled from the abdomen under visual control. If there is no bleeding from these 5 mm port sites, no fascial or skin sutures are placed. However, in a prepubertal child, the fascia of even the 5 mm port sites should be closed. In the male patient, if a pneumoscrotum has developed during the procedure, the scrotum is manually decompressed.

If any bleeding is noted coming from a trocar incision site, either electrocoagulation of the site or placement of an 0 absorbable suture is necessary. To determine in which quadrant a vessel has been injured, the trocar can be cantilevered in each of four directions: superiorly, inferiorly, medially, and laterally. Pressure on the abdominal wall in one of these four directions should momentarily stop the bleeding; it is across this quadrant that the hemostatic suture is placed. The suture encompasses the entire thickness of the abdominal wall. This can be done in one of two ways. A large curved needle (BP-48, taper) or a straight Keith needle on an 0 absorbable suture is passed, under endoscopic monitoring, directly into the abdominal cavity. If the abdominal wall is thin, a through-and-through transperitoneal suture can be secured with one pass of the large curved needle.

If the patient is not thin, a Keith needle is used. The point of entry should be just inferior to the probable site of bleeding. Once seen in the abdomen, the straight needle can be grasped with a 5 mm laparoscopic needle holder and passed inside out of the abdomen just superior to the probable site of bleeding (Fig. 11-3, *A*). The laparoscopic sheath is removed. The suture is secured by tying it down on a rolled gauze pad or other type of bolster (Fig. 11-3, *B*). If done correctly, there should be no further bleeding from the site of the peritoneotomy.

Alternatively, or if sutures do not control hemorrhage from the port site, the sheath is removed and a Foley catheter with a 30 cc balloon is inserted into the peritoneal cavity. The balloon is inflated and the cath-

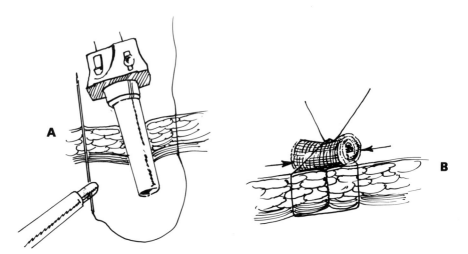

Fig. 11-3 **A,** Keith needle is used to traverse the suspected site of bleeding. **B,** The 5 mm sheath is removed and the suture is tied over a gauze bolster.

eter is pulled anteriorly while monitoring the intra-abdominal appearance via the laparoscope. With appropriate traction, bleeding from vessels in the abdominal wall will be arrested with this maneuver. The catheter is anchored at the skin level with a Kelly clamp overnight, after which the balloon is deflated and the catheter removed.

The last sheath to be removed is the 5 mm sheath through which the 5 mm laparoscope has been passed (Fig. 11-4). At this point one of two methods of desufflation may be followed. In the first technique, the pneumoperitoneum is maintained by having the assistant place a finger over each of the other 5 mm port sites. The last 5 mm sheath is slowly backed out of the abdomen with the tip of the 5 mm laparoscope protruding beyond the end of the sheath (see Fig. 11-4). As the 5 mm laparoscope is withdrawn, the sites of the peritoneotomy and fasciotomy are inspected to rule out bleeding.

Alternatively, after the other sheaths have been removed, the abdominal wall surrounding the last sheath may be manually lifted. With the port still just barely in the peritoneal cavity, the sidearm is opened and the CO_2 in the abdomen is allowed to escape. Active ventilation at this time is also helpful. When the abdomen is desufflated, the 5 mm laparoscope is introduced to push any bowel away from the tip of the

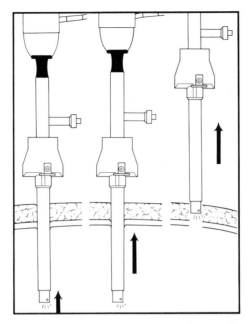

Fig. 11-4 As the last sheath is removed, the tract is inspected for bleeding. Throughout this maneuver, the laparoscope protrudes beyond the tip of the sheath.

sheath. The tip of the laparoscope should extend slightly beyond the end of the sheath. The sheath and laparoscope are then withdrawn as a unit and the peritoneotomy and fasciotomy sites are inspected for bleeding.

If bleeding is noted from the final 5 mm port site, and if it is at the superficial muscle or skin level, then the site is electrocoagulated; if this fails, an 0 absorbable suture is placed as described in the previous paragraph. In this case, it is necessary to maintain or reestablish the pneumoperitoneum and to replace the 5 mm laparoscope through one of the other 5 mm sites to monitor the placement and effect of the suture. Again, this is necessary only in the rare circumstance that the surgeon notes blood coming from the last 5 mm port site.

Finally, the skin site of all ports is closed with an adhesive strip. With this method of exiting the abdomen, no bowel or omentum should become entrapped by the fascial sutures, nor should herniation occur through any of the port sites.

PAIN CONTROL

Near the completion of a laparoscopic procedure, postoperative pain management may be aided by intramuscular or intravenous injection of a nonsteroidal anti-inflammatory agent such as ketorolac tromethamine (Toradol). Ideally this is given approximately 30 minutes before completion of the procedure. In addition, injection of a local anesthetic such as 0.25% bupivacaine (Marcaine) with epinephrine into the abdominal incisions may minimize postoperative incisional discomfort.

TROUBLESHOOTING

Problem: Pneumoscrotum.
Solution: Manual decompression.

Problem: Acute "hydrocele."
Solution: Observation, reassurance.

Problem: Abdominal wall bleeding from a trocar site.
Solution: Circular suture of full thickness of abdominal wall done with a curved or Keith needle (see Fig. 11-3) or Foley catheter tamponade.

CHAPTER 12

Postoperative Care

David M. Albala and Ralph V. Clayman

General Care
Medications
Convalescence
Troubleshooting

GENERAL CARE

For simple laparoscopic procedures with a low risk of significant complications and requiring less than an hour to complete (e.g., liver biopsy, inguinal hernia repair, tubal ligation, diagnostic laparoscopy), the patient can usually be discharged to home on an outpatient basis after monitoring in the recovery room (Appendix B). Lengthier and more extensive procedures usually require anywhere from an overnight to a 5-day hospital stay.

The patient is ambulated 2 to 3 hours after the procedure. If the intestinal tract has not been opened, oral intake is usually started when the patient returns to the outpatient area or to his or her hospital bed. The diet is advanced as tolerated to a regular diet, usually by the evening of the same day as the procedure or by the next morning.

MEDICATIONS

Medications during the postoperative period usually consist of an analgesic and antibiotic. Narcotic analgesics may be needed during the initial 24 hours following laparoscopy; after that period Tylenol should suffice. For painful postoperative diaphragmatic irritation, a 30 to 60 mg intramuscular loading dose of ketorolac tromethamine (Toradol) is quite effective, followed by 15 to 30 mg intramuscularly every 6 hours as needed. This may be continued orally: 10 mg every 4 to 6 hours as needed. When narcotic analgesics are needed beyond 24 hours or when the patient's discomfort begins to increase 24 hours after the procedure, he or she should be evaluated for a possible unrecognized bowel perforation.

Antibiotics are needed only for 24 to 36 hours after the procedure, if at all. Usually one additional dose of a parenteral antibiotic in the postoperative period is sufficient. There is no need to discharge the patient on a regimen of oral antibiotics. The adhesive skin strips can be removed in 1 week.

CONVALESCENCE

Full convalescence should occur in 2 to 14 days, depending on the extent of the procedure. When the patient is discharged within 24 hours of a therapeutic laparoscopic procedure, he or she should be made aware that abdominal wall edema or ecchymoses may develop at home. Albeit visually impressive, this is usually of no clinical significance and resolves within a few weeks.

The surgeon should be aware that some of the complications of a laparoscopic procedure may not appear literally for months postoperatively. Indeed, some postoperative lymphoceles, infected pelvic hematomas, and a bowel perforation have each occurred more than 3 months after an apparently routine laparoscopic pelvic lymph node dissection.

TROUBLESHOOTING

Problem: Abdominal pain.

Solution: If the abdominal pain is localized to a port site, the differential diagnosis includes *localized* infection or herniation. The first condition occurs 1 to 2 weeks postoperatively and is readily recognized; treatment is incision, drainage, and oral antibiotics. For herniation through one of the larger port sites (i.e., ≥10 mm), the procedure to reduce the hernia can be performed laparoscopically. The hernia sac can be cleanly dissected from the old port site, and this site can then be sutured closed from the inside of the abdomen.

If the abdominal pain is *diffuse*, the patient may have a bowel obstruction caused by adhesions or may have an unrecognized bowel injury that occurred at the time of the laparoscopic procedure. This will require open exploration. Remember, generalized peritonitis remains one of the contraindications to any laparoscopic procedure.

Problem: Postoperative hydrocele.
Solution: In male patients undergoing laparoscopic procedures, especially hernia repair or pelvic lymph node dissection, any irrigating
fluid used during the procedure may accumulate in the scrotum. This
may not be noticeable until the patient is ambulatory. The hydrocele
can be quite massive and require additional bed rest and the use of
a scrotal support. It resolves spontaneously over a 7- to 14-day period.

Problem: Lower limb edema.
Solution: After pelvic lymphadenectomy, mild lower limb edema may
develop. The only treatment is use of support hose. In these patients
the surgeon should order a pelvic CT scan to rule out the possibility
that the lymphedema is secondary to a postoperative pelvic mass
(i.e., hematoma or lymphocele). If the lower extremity edema is bilateral, other systemic causes, in addition to the local problems,
should be ruled out (e.g., fluid overload, congestive heart failure).

Problem: Abdominal wall ecchymoses.
Solution: This problem can be quite impressive; indeed, the scrotum
and entire lower half of the abdomen may become ecchymotic following a laparoscopic groin operation. The full visual impact of this
problem is usually not apparent until after the patient has been discharged from the hospital. If the patient is having no discomfort and
the hematocrit level is unchanged, then reassurance is all that is
necessary. This condition will usually resolve spontaneously over the
ensuing 2 to 3 weeks.

However, if the development of abdominal wall ecchymosis is
accompanied by discomfort or a fall in the hematocrit level, this may
represent delayed hemorrhage and a CT scan of the abdomen is
indicated to rule out the possibility of a developing intrapelvic hematoma. If delayed active bleeding is suspected, a labeled red blood
cell study or angiogram may be helpful to identify the site of the
hemorrhage. If the bleeding is from one of the branches of the iliac
vein or artery, percutaneous embolization can be performed. Failing
this approach, an open exploration, with a vascular surgeon present,
is necessary.

Problem: Delayed abdominal or pelvic discomfort.
Solution: As long as 3 to 5 months after the primary laparoscopic procedure, the patient may present with vague lower quadrant abdominal discomfort. An abdominal-pelvic CT scan should be performed.
To date, there have been occurrences of late presentations of lymphoceles, infected pelvic hematomas, and even a bowel fistula.

Problem: Severe shoulder pain of pleuritic nature.

Prevention: Evacuate CO_2 from abdomen at the end of the procedure (see Chapter 11).

Solution: When this occurs in the immediate postoperative period, it is probably diaphragmatic irritation from CO_2. This type of discomfort responds rapidly to ketorolac tromethamine (30 to 60 mg intramuscular loading dose, followed by 15 to 30 mg every 6 hours as needed). Usually only 1 to 2 doses are needed.

However, because of the length of many laparoscopic procedures, an arterial blood gas determination and ventilation/perfusion scan may be obtained in these patients to rule out a pulmonary embolus; an ECG is performed to rule out any cardiac problems that might present with diaphragmatic symptoms.

CHAPTER 13

Complications of Laparoscopy
Strategies for Prevention and Treatment

William A. See, Terri G. Monk, and B. Craig Weldon

Laparoscopic surgery, when performed by the experienced surgeon, is remarkably free of significant complications. The overall incidence of complications related to laparoscopy is 4%, with a mortality rate of 0.03%.[1,2] The surgical team must have a complete understanding of the pathophysiology of laparoscopic complications and their clinical manifestations. This knowledge can radically improve the outcome of even the most adverse events by facilitating their early diagnosis and treatment. In this chapter intraoperative and postoperative laparoscopic complications will be examined from the perspective of their prevention, diagnosis, and treatment (see the box on p. 217).

INTRAOPERATIVE COMPLICATIONS

Intraoperative complications include those associated with anesthesia and those related to the laparoscopic technique. The majority of problems involve the cardiovascular and pulmonary systems. Vascular, neurologic, and visceral injuries are rare but potentially serious complications.[3]

Cardiovascular complications
Gas embolus

Problem   Carbon dioxide (CO_2) is the gas most commonly used to establish a pneumoperitoneum for laparoscopy because it is highly soluble in blood and nonflammable.[3,4] The lethal intravenous dose of CO_2 in dogs is five times greater than that of injected room air (i.e., 5 ml/kg air versus 25 ml/kg CO_2).[5] The high blood solubility of CO_2 allows it to be rapidly absorbed into the bloodstream and exhaled via the lungs. Nitrous oxide is nearly as soluble as CO_2 in plasma (60% to 80% of the solubility of CO_2).[4]

Venous gas embolism is a potential, catastrophic cause of cardiovascular collapse during laparoscopy.[6-12] This is usually secondary to inadvertent placement of the Veress needle into a blood vessel or vascular organ. When a critical volume of gas reaches the right ventricle, it creates an "air lock" in the pulmonary outflow tract that impedes pulmonary circulation.[13] A high-grade obstruction to pulmonary blood flow rapidly leads to right ventricular failure with a catastrophic drop in pulmonary venous flow and left ventricular output.

Prevention   Careful placement of the Veress needle with appropriate safety measures (see Chapter 8) before insufflation and use of CO_2 and not air, for insufflation should markedly reduce the incidence of this complication.

Diagnosis   Capnometry, with end-tidal CO_2 monitoring, allows an early diagnosis of venous gas embolism. This event causes a precipitous fall in the end-tidal CO_2 concentration (within a few breaths) because

Laparoscopic principles of problem prevention

1. Patient selection
   Identify high-risk patients
2. Informed consent
   Include the possibility of open surgical intervention
3. Patient preparation
   Type and screen or cross-match (2 units) for blood products
   Instill perioperative antibiotics
   Include capnometry, pulse oximetry, and continuous ECG with standard
      monitors
   Secure and appropriately pad patient
   Insert nasogastric or orogastric tube
   Insert Foley urethral catheter
   Full abdominal skin preparation
4. Properly maintained equipment
   Sharp trocars
   Appropriately shielded electrosurgical instruments
5. Working knowledge of equipment
   Insufflator
   Irrigator/aspirator
6. Standardized approach to performing the procedure
   Assess Veress needle placement
   Monitor insufflation pressure
   Establish adequate pneumoperitoneum
   Prevent uncontrolled excursion of trocars
   Transilluminate abdominal wall to avoid injury to superficial abdominal
      vessels during secondary trocar placement
   Visually monitor insertion of all secondary trocars
   Inspect abdominal contents for potential injury
   Intermittently monitor pneumoperitoneum pressure
   Inspect all trocar insertion sites at the start and completion of the pro-
      cedure to exclude unrecognized visceral injury or active bleeding, re-
      spectively
   Close fascia of ≥10 mm trocar insertion sites
7. Establish a consistent laparoscopy team with experienced surgical assistant
   and scrub nurse

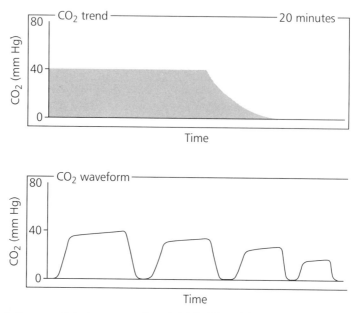

Fig. 13-1 Exponential decrease of end-tidal CO_2. This pattern usually signals a catastrophic event—that is, cardiopulmonary arrest, severe pulmonary hypoperfusion, or gas embolus.

of the acute loss of pulmonary perfusion (Fig. 13-1). Auscultation of a "mill wheel" murmur over the precordium, a sudden decline in oxygen saturation, and profound hypotension are also signs associated with a gas embolus.

Treatment In addition to general resuscitative efforts, treatment of gas embolism includes cessation of insufflation, immediate release of the pneumoperitoneum (i.e., desufflation), and placement of the patient in a steep, head-down left lateral decubitus (i.e., left-side-down/right-side-up) position to minimize the right ventricular outflow tract obstruction (Fig. 13-2). Attempts should also be made to aspirate gas from the right side of the heart following advancement of the central venous pressure (CVP) catheter. If a pulmonary artery (PA) catheter is in place, it is reasonable to attempt to aspirate gas through both the PA and CVP ports. However, aspiration of embolized gas via a pulmonary artery catheter is reported to be less successful than aspiration via a CVP catheter.[14]

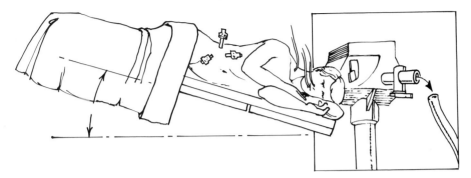

Fig. 13-2 Acute management of gas embolus: the pneumoperitoneum is released (inset), and the patient is immediately placed in a head-down, right-side-up (i.e., left lateral decubitus) position.

Hypotension

Problem Hypotension during laparoscopy may result from a decrease in venous return, reduced cardiac output, or a drop in circulating blood volume. Insufflation of gas into the peritoneal cavity results in an increase in intra-abdominal pressure and vena caval compression with subsequent reduction in venous return to the heart.[15-18] Insufflation to intra-abdominal pressures of 20 mm Hg is routinely well tolerated; however, increases in intra-abdominal pressure >30 mm Hg often decrease cardiac output and arterial blood pressure.[17,18] Other less common causes of hypotension include bradycardia secondary to vagal stimulation, hypoxia, venous gas embolism, pneumothorax, and anesthetic overdose.

Prevention To maintain adequate venous return, the intra-abdominal pressure should remain ≤15 mm Hg. In many situations a pressure of 10 mm Hg provides sufficient abdominal distention and adequate venous return. Circulating blood volume must be maintained in a normal range throughout surgery.

Diagnosis A decrease in systolic arterial blood pressure greater than 20% to 30% below the patient's normal blood pressure range represents hypotension. However, organ ischemia may develop in patients with severe cardiovascular or central nervous system problems if their blood pressure is allowed to fall below their "normal" values. Thus the anesthesiologist must determine the acceptable intraoperative blood pressure range for each patient.

Treatment The management of hypotensive emergencies includes immediate release of the pneumoperitoneum (i.e., desufflation to restore intra-abdominal pressure to 0 mm Hg), decrease in anesthetic concentrations, and rapid administration of intravenous fluid. In addition, the patient should be placed in the head-down position to increase venous return. If auscultation of the chest indicates a pneumothorax, immediate tube thoracostomy is necessary; if a gas embolus is suspected, the patient is kept head-down but also turned into a left lateral decubitus position (see Fig. 13-2). For bradycardia secondary to vagal stimulation, 0.4 to 0.8 mg of atropine given intravenously is the recommended treatment. The addition of vasopressors (i.e., ephedrine, 5 to 10 mg/dose intravenously; or phenylephrine, 50 to 100 μg/dose intravenously) may also be necessary to correct hypotension.

Hypertension

Problem Absorption of CO_2 and subsequent hypercarbia may stimulate the sympathetic nervous system, resulting in tachycardia and hypertension.[19] Inadequate depth of anesthesia and hypoxia may also cause elevations in blood pressure. Intraoperative hypertension is more common in patients with a history of essential hypertension.[20]

Prevention It is important to continue current antihypertensive therapy throughout the perioperative period in all patients with essential hypertension. This includes administration of antihypertensive medication on the morning of surgery. Also, keeping the intra-abdominal pressure at ≤15 mm Hg helps to prevent hypercarbia. The anesthesiologist must diligently monitor the patient's ventilation, oxygenation, and depth of anesthesia during the procedure.

Diagnosis Noninvasive blood pressure monitoring is routine during all surgical procedures. Invasive monitoring with an intra-arterial catheter is indicated in patients with poorly controlled blood pressure preoperatively. The patient's preoperative blood pressure is used as a guide to determine his or her "safe" intraoperative blood pressure range. As a guideline we consider blood pressure elevations of 20% to 30% above the patient's normal range or a diastolic blood pressure ≥100 mm Hg as representing intraoperative hypertension.

Treatment The initial management of hypertension should be directed at increasing the patient's ventilation (if hypercarbia is present) and increasing the depth of anesthesia. The inspired oxygen concentration should be increased to provide adequate oxygenation. Vasodilatory agents (i.e., nitroglycerin, sodium nitroprusside) are popular for intraoperative blood pressure control because of their rapid onset and short duration. The α- or β-adrenergic blocking agents (i.e., phentolamine, labetalol, propanolol) can also be added for blood pressure control.

Arrhythmias

Problem   Cardiac arrhythmias occur in 25% to 47% of patients during laparoscopic surgery.[21-23] *Bradyarrhythmias* occur in 30% of women during CO_2 insufflation or traction on pelvic structures[6] and may on rare occasions progress to sinus arrest.[8,24,25] Hypercarbia from systemic absorption of CO_2 frequently produces *sinus tachycardia* and *premature ventricular contractions*, although venous gas embolus, hypoxia, and inadequate anesthetic level must also be considered in the differential diagnosis of these arrhythmias.[3,21,23,25]

Prevention   It is important to maintain the pneumoperitoneum at ≤15 mm Hg and avoid hypercarbia (i.e., maintain the end-tidal CO_2 ≤45 mm Hg).

Diagnosis   Monitoring the heart's electrical activity with an ECG is a routine anesthetic practice. Cardiac arrhythmias are readily detected by close observation of the ECG.

Treatment   The initial treatment of cardiac arrhythmias during laparoscopy includes reduction of the intra-abdominal pressure (i.e., desufflation), release of traction on any pelvic organs, and hyperventilation with 100% oxygen. Proper positioning of the endotracheal tube and adequate oxygenation must be ensured. Persistent bradycardia may require treatment with 0.4 to 0.8 mg of intravenous atropine to prevent progression to cardiac arrest. Ventricular arrhythmias may be treated with lidocaine, 0.5 to 1.0 mg/kg intravenously, followed by an infusion of 2 to 4 mg/min.

Monitoring artifacts

Problem   Clinical measurement of CVP and pulmonary artery pressure (PAP) actually reflects the sum of the intravascular pressure plus pleural pressure.[16] Increased inspiratory inflation pressures are needed to provide adequate ventilation during abdominal insufflation. Thus CVP or PAP may be falsely elevated by the increased pleural pressures and may not accurately reflect venous return and cardiac output during laparoscopy.

Prevention   Intra-abdominal pressure should remain ≤15 mm Hg during laparoscopy to avoid the need for elevated inspiratory inflation pressures.

Diagnosis   Monitoring the aneroid pressure gauge in the breathing circuit during insufflation is mandatory. If inflation pressure increases, the CVP or PAP measurement will reflect the elevation in pleural pressure.

Treatment   Do not rely on the CVP or PAP to accurately reflect venous return or cardiac function during laparoscopy. If an accurate assessment of these parameters is desired, direct measurement of cardiac output is necessary. Transesophageal echocardiography can also be used to monitor volume status and cardiac function.

Pulmonary complications
Hypoxemia

Problem   Ventilation-perfusion mismatching is a major cause of hypoxemia during laparoscopy. Its cause is multifactorial. First, the head-down position causes the weight of the abdominal contents to rest on the diaphragm,[26] which subsequently decreases lung volume and contributes to the development of atelectasis, especially in the elderly, obese, or debilitated patient.[27,28] In addition, the head-down position displaces the lungs and carina upward while the endotracheal tube is fixed, thereby creating the potential for migration of the endotracheal tube from the trachea into a main-stem bronchus.[28] Third, the head-down position results in pooling of blood in dependent portions of the lungs, which further worsens ventilation-perfusion abnormalities.[29] Finally, insufflation to intra-abdominal pressures of 25 mm Hg exerts a force of approximately 30 g/cm^2 (total pressure of 50 kg) against the diaphragm, which further restricts lung expansion and decreases pulmonary compliance.[22]

Prevention   It may be necessary to increase the minute ventilation during controlled ventilation to compensate for the pulmonary changes that develop following positioning of the patient and establishment of the pneumoperitoneum.

Diagnosis   The development of intraoperative ventilation-perfusion abnormalities is suggested if the patient's oxygen saturation declines as measured by pulse oximetry or the patient requires increased inspiratory inflation pressures to maintain minute ventilation at a constant level.[30]

Treatment   Derangements in oxygenation and/or ventilation should be treated with hyperventilation with 100% oxygen, elimination of the head-down position, release of the pneumoperitoneum (i.e., desufflation), and auscultation of the chest to verify the position of the endotracheal tube and to rule out a pneumothorax.

Hypercarbia/acidosis

Problem Hypercarbia is usually secondary to absorption of insufflated CO_2 into the vascular system or to ventilation-perfusion mismatching during the procedure.[1,3,17,18,30-33] When local or epidural anesthesia with light sedation is used for laparoscopy, patients increase their minute ventilation to maintain a normal $PaCO_2$.[32,33] Also, during general anesthesia, patients who are allowed to breathe spontaneously have a significantly higher $PaCO_2$ compared with patients with controlled ventilation.[30] The physiologic effects of hypercarbia include autonomic stimulation of the cardiovascular system (i.e., tachycardia, hypertension) followed by acidosis-mediated myocardial depression, vasodilation, and hypotension.

Prevention Currently efforts are being made to investigate alternative insufflation gases (e.g., helium) for laparoscopy or to create the working space by using devices that elevate the abdominal wall actively, thereby eliminating the need to expand the abdominal cavity with CO_2.

Diagnosis Capnometry will detect the onset of hypercarbia; therefore monitoring of end-tidal CO_2 is essential during laparoscopy (Fig. 13-3). The end-tidal CO_2 should be maintained between 30 and 40 mm Hg, which usually ensures that the $PaCO_2$ is ≤50 mm Hg. However, in

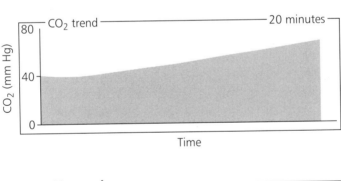

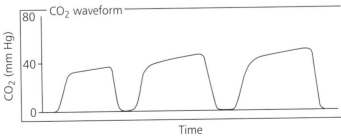

Fig. 13-3 Gradual increase of end-tidal CO_2. This may be associated with CO_2 absorption resulting from high insufflation pressures, hypoventilation, or partial airway obstruction.

patients with ventilation-perfusion abnormalities (i.e., chronic obstructive pulmonary disease), the end-tidal CO_2 will grossly underestimate the $PaCO_2$. Thus periodic arterial blood gas sampling (i.e., every 1 to 2 hours) to determine arterial pH, $PaCO_2$, and PaO_2 is recommended.

Treatment If hypercarbia occurs, the minute ventilation can be increased while the surgeon desufflates the abdomen and the patient is moved to a "head-up" position. Further insufflation of CO_2 must await resolution of the hypercarbia. When the procedure is resumed, the pneumoperitoneum should be maintained at a lower insufflation pressure if feasible (e.g., 10 mm Hg).

Aspiration

Problem Both head-down positioning and increased intra-abdominal pressure predispose the anesthetized patient to regurgitation and aspiration of gastric contents.[34,35] Kurer and Welch[36] reported that intraoperative aspiration does not occur in young, nonobese women undergoing laparoscopic procedures of less than 20 minutes' duration. However, many laparoscopic procedures exceed 20 minutes and are not performed on healthy, nonobese patients.

Prevention If a lengthy procedure is anticipated or the risk for aspiration is high (e.g., in a morbidly obese patient), then general anesthesia with endotracheal intubation using a *cuffed* endotracheal tube is the best way to preclude this problem. Also, the routine placement of a nasogastric tube for the duration of lengthier procedures further reduces the chances of aspiration.

Diagnosis Aspiration should be considered if vomiting or regurgitation occurs before endotracheal intubation. Clinical signs of aspiration include wheezing, tachypnea, laryngospasm, bronchospasm, hypoxemia, coughing, tachycardia, and hypotension. The radiographic picture may show lobar consolidation (right lower lobe is the most common location) or fluffy infiltrates.

Treatment If the findings suggest aspiration, the patient should be intubated and the trachea suctioned before initiating ventilation of the lungs. Positive pressure ventilation with 100% oxygen should be instituted to prevent atelectasis and hypoxia. The surgery should be delayed until the severity of the aspiration is evaluated. Prophylactic treatment with antibiotics or steroids is not recommended.[37]

Pneumothorax

Problem A pneumothorax can occur if (1) defects in the diaphragm allow the insufflating gas to pass into the thoracic cavity,[38-41] (2) positive pressure ventilation causes barotrauma to the lung, or (3) a trocar is placed above the twelfth rib.[42]

Prevention Laterally placed trocars should not be positioned intercostally. Intra-abdominal pressure should remain ≤15 mm Hg throughout the procedure.

Diagnosis Small amounts of air in the pleural space may not cause symptoms. However, a tension pneumothorax is accompanied by a unilateral decrease in breath sounds, wheezing, progressive tracheal deviation, hypotension, and an increase in ventilatory pressure. A chest x-ray film, with the patient upright if possible, will confirm the diagnosis.

Treatment A pneumothorax of ≤20% can be treated expectantly. However, positive pressure ventilation usually expands a pneumothorax and may lead to cardiovascular compromise (tension pneumothorax). If cardiovascular collapse is imminent, the involved hemithorax should be punctured with a large-bore needle. The needle is inserted above the rib in the midclavicular line of the second or third intercostal space. A tube thoracostomy is then performed in the fourth intercostal space just behind the anterior axillary fold with a 24 to 28 Fr chest tube. Immediately following placement, the chest tube is connected to water seal and suction; proper chest tube placement is verified with a chest x-ray film.[43] Whenever a pneumothorax is suspected, nitrous oxide administration should be terminated, because this gas will diffuse into a pneumothorax and rapidly expand its volume.

Pneumomediastinum/pneumopericardium

Problem During laparoscopy, gas may enter the thorax via congenital defects or weak points in the diaphragm.[39] The air then dissects along the blood vessels toward the mediastinum, resulting in a pneumomediastinum and/or pneumopericardium.[38]

Prevention This problem can be minimized by slow insufflation of gas and maintenance of intra-abdominal pressure ≤15 mm Hg.

Diagnosis These complications should be considered if subcutaneous emphysema or pneumothorax occurs. Pneumomediastinum is rarely associated with adverse physiologic effects. Pneumopericardium, on the other hand, has the potential for causing a major deterioration of cardiovascular function. The diagnosis is confirmed by the presence of air in the mediastinum or pericardium on a chest radiograph.

Treatment Pneumomediastinum may be a harbinger of impending pneumothorax and mandates immediate release of the pneumoperitoneum. Careful consideration should be given to terminating the surgical procedure to avoid the development of serious complications. Most cases of pneumomediastinum/pneumopericardium will resolve spontaneously with observation and supportive therapy.[38] However, if the pneumopericardium results in a pericardial tamponade, pericardiocentesis may be necessary.

Miscellaneous complications
Subcutaneous emphysema/properitoneal insufflation

Problem   Subcutaneous CO_2 emphysema can occur at any time between the initiation of the pneumoperitoneum and the removal of the insufflating cannula. Common causes for this problem include improper placement of the Veress needle, leakage of CO_2 around trocars, and malfunction of or improper use of the CO_2 insufflator.[37,38]

Likewise, if the Veress needle is beneath the subcutaneous tissue but has not pierced the peritoneum, then properitoneal insufflation may occur. The properitoneal placement of the Veress needle makes correct needle placement much more difficult. Gaseous expansion of the properitoneal space effectively reduces the volume of the peritoneal cavity and increases the distance that the Veress needle must travel to enter the peritoneal cavity (Fig. 13-4, *A*). Also, the surgeon should be aware that properitoneal insufflation may cause significant stretching of the peritoneum and an associated vasovagal reaction.

Prevention   To avoid this problem, correct initial Veress needle placement, or early recognition of incorrect placement, is essential. A number of maneuvers can be used to increase the likelihood of correct needle placement. Two distinct "pops" or "clicks" of the Veress needle should be heard or felt as the needle first traverses the anterior abdominal wall fascia and then traverses the peritoneal membrane. Placing a small drop of sterile saline or water on the hub of the Veress needle (i.e., *drop test*) will allow visualization of the negative pressure encountered if the abdominal cavity has been entered; the negative intra-abdominal pressure occurring during respiration should cause the drop of fluid to be sucked into the barrel of the needle.

An additional step that is essential in the identification of incorrect needle placement is the *aspiration and saline injection test*. Once the Veress needle is felt to be in the correct location, it is connected to a 10 ml syringe and suction is applied. No fluid should be drawn into the barrel of the syringe. A fluid return suggests needle placement in bowel (yellow or brown fluid), bladder (clear or yellow fluid), or a vascular structure. Provided no fluid returns at the time of the initial aspiration, 10 ml of saline should next be injected through the needle. If the needle

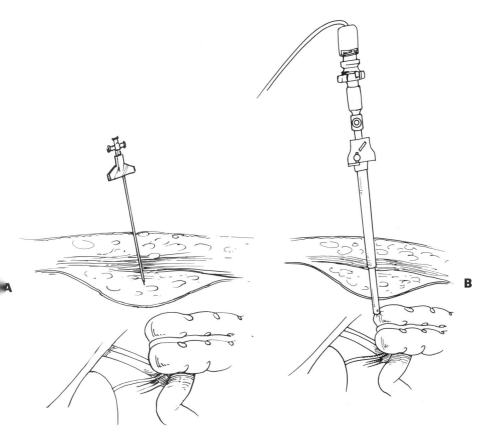

Fig. 13-4 **A,** Properitoneal insufflation. **B,** Anterior displacement of the sheath into the properitoneal space; as the properitoneum fills with CO_2, the surgeons intra-abdominal view decreases despite having the laparoscope in the abdomen.

lies within the peritoneal cavity, the saline should flow easily and attempts to aspirate any of the instilled saline should be unsuccessful. If the needle lies in the properitoneal space, then while the saline may still be instilled without much resistance, aspiration usually results in the return of several milliliters of saline, thereby indicating the properitoneal position of the Veress needle.

Also at this time, an advancement test can be performed; if the Veress needle is truly in the peritoneal cavity, it can be advanced 1 to 2 cm deeper without encountering any resistance. However, if the needle lies in the properitoneal space, the same advancement will encounter resistance from the peritoneum, indicating that the needle is still too superficial.

The next most important indicator of correct needle positioning is the initial insufflation pressure when establishing the pneumoperitoneum. Initial insufflation pressures <10 mm Hg are typical of correct placement. Starting pressures >10 mm Hg warrant removal and reinsertion of the Veress needle. Occasionally increased pressures result from the needle lumen abutting an intra-abdominal structure. Needle rotation will help to exclude this possibility. If the intra-abdominal pressures are still >10 mm Hg despite needle rotation, the needle should be immediately withdrawn and the insertion procedure repeated. The decision to maintain or remove the Veress needle should be made before 250 ml of CO_2 is insufflated. Proper positioning of the Veress needle is an "all or none" phenomenon: "When in doubt, pull it out."

If the needle is correctly positioned, initial CO_2 insufflation at 1 L/min flow should result in a symmetrically distended abdominal cavity. Also, after 1 L of CO_2 is insufflated, percussion over the liver should reveal tympany.

Diagnosis The insufflation pressures are usually >10 mm Hg, and high pressures occur with <1 L of CO_2 insufflated. If the Veress needle is in the subcutaneous tissue, then crepitus develops over the abdomen and thorax. However, if the Veress needle lies properitoneally, then, in male patients, a pneumoscrotum may develop.

Delayed recognition of properitoneal insufflation normally occurs at the time of primary trocar insertion. Minimal CO_2 return, combined with visualization of only fat when inserting the laparoscope, is characteristic of the problem.

Similarly, if properitoneal insufflation develops during the procedure, the sheath may have been inadvertently retracted. When this occurs, the sheath will lie in the properitoneal space unbeknownst to the surgeon, since the laparoscope has been passed through the sheath and still lies in the abdomen (Fig. 13-4, *B*).

Treatment When properitoneal insufflation is noted at the time of primary trocar placement, courses of action include abandoning the laparoscopic approach, a minilaparotomy trocar insertion using the open cannula, or repeat attempts at creating a pneumoperitoneum using the Veress needle placed under endoscopic monitoring. Alternatively, one can try to allow the CO_2 to escape and begin anew at the same or a different site. In the latter circumstance, in a female patient, a transfundal or cul de sac approach may work well.

Intraoperatively the problem of subcutaneous emphysema may be overcome by (1) repositioning the Veress needle, (2) checking insufflator function, (3) placing a purse-string suture/petrolatum gauze around any leaking trocar site, (4) replacing a "leaking" trocar with a larger trocar, and/or (5) sliding the sheath through which the laparoscope has been passed deeper into the peritoneal cavity.

At the end of a laparoscopic procedure, subcutaneous or properitoneal emphysema generally requires no specific intervention, because this situation rapidly resolves following the completion of the procedure and cessation of insufflation. Likewise, a pneumopenis or pneumoscrotum can be resolved by manually expressing the CO_2 from these structures at the end of the procedure.

Vascular injury

Problem   Vascular injuries most often occur during Veress needle or primary (i.e., "blind") trocar placement. The severity of vascular injuries ranges from insignificant hematoma formation in the abdominal wall to laceration of the abdominal aorta.[1,37]

The aorta, inferior vena cava, and right common iliac vessels have the greatest potential for life-threatening injury from umbilical access.

Prevention   There are many precautions the surgeon can take to prevent vascular injury during initial "blind" trocar passage. First, by nicking the fascia with a knife, resistance to trocar passage can be greatly reduced. Next, the middle finger of the dominant trocar-wielding hand should be extended down the shaft of the trocar to serve as a brake, thereby precluding a sudden deep passage of the trocar. The use of a "new" sharp trocar equipped with a locking safety shield is helpful. Furthermore, the entire trocar sheath and safety shield should clear the incision site before any forceful efforts are made to pass the trocar into the abdomen. Next, the surgeon and the first assistant can stabilize the abdominal wall by placing a towel clip on either side of the trocar site. This will prevent the downward motion of the abdominal wall as the trocar is pushed forward. By transiently raising the intra-abdominal pressure to 25 mm Hg, additional CO_2 can be instilled into the abdomen, thereby pushing the peritoneum more firmly against the anterior abdominal wall and increasing the cushion of CO_2 between the anterior abdominal wall and the retroperitoneal vascular structures.

Transillumination of the abdominal wall before secondary trocar passage can help the surgeon to identify superficial abdominal wall vessels and thus avoid injuring them with either a knife or trocar. In performing this maneuver, the surgeon must remember to change the light setting on the light source from video to manual; the room lights must be turned off.

Also, constant *visual* monitoring of placement of all secondary trocars is essential. Specifically, when inserting lateral trocars, if the inferior epigastric vessels are "seen" as they course along the anterior abdominal wall, they can be avoided and chances of trocar injury can be significantly decreased.

All instruments must be endoscopically tracked as they are passed into the operative field. No instrument should be opened and closed unless it is under direct endoscopic monitoring.

By lowering the intra-abdominal pressure to 5 mm Hg at the end of the procedure, any significant venous injuries should become apparent. Trocar removal must be done under direct visual monitoring at 5 mm Hg to rule out any bleeding from the abdominal wall trocar sites.

Diagnosis Puncture of a large vessel (i.e., aorta) is rapidly evident because the withdrawal of the obturator is accompanied by a gush of blood. Injury to smaller vessels may produce a constant dripping of blood into the abdominal cavity along the sleeve of a secondary trocar.

Unfortunately, the presentation of a retroperitoneal trocar vascular injury may not be immediately obvious. In this situation, the retroperitoneal space fills with blood, thereby reducing the size of the space within the peritoneal cavity. Despite a pneumoperitoneum that registers 15 mm Hg, the surgeon "feels" that the "field" is closing. The next sign may be the onset of hemodynamic instability. Indeed, occult hemorrhage should always be foremost in the surgeon's mind whenever there are significant changes in the patient's vital signs, either intraoperatively or in the recovery room.

Similarly, injuries from blind instrument passage may be difficult to recognize and may be seen as a gradual accumulation of blood in the peritoneal cavity or operative field from an "unrecognized" site.

Treatment The potential for rapid blood loss mandates that every patient undergoing laparoscopic surgery have the full field of the abdomen prepared and draped and a large-bore intravenous line placed. In addition, a type and screen or a cross-match for 2 units of blood should be done before any extensive laparoscopic therapeutic procedure. *An open laparotomy set must be immediately available in the OR during ALL laparoscopic procedures.*

Bleeding at the level of the abdominal wall can be managed by combined external/laparoscopic suture ligation. In contrast, attempts at direct laparoscopic control of intra-abdominal vascular injuries should be limited to relatively small vessels that are directly accessible and not an immediate threat to the patient's hemodynamic stability. Electrosurgery, Nd:YAG or KTP laser, clips, ligature loops, and argon beam coagulation constitute the laparoscopic armamentarium available for non-life-threatening vascular control. Unfortunately, the rapid accumulation of blood in the dependent locations in which many significant vascular injuries occur, together with the limited suction/irrigation capability of most available instruments, limits laparoscopic vascular repair.

When bleeding is encountered during laparoscopic dissection, the tip of the laparoscope may initially become covered with blood. The immediate concern is that the bleeding is significant; however, this is usually not the case. The surgeon should remove the laparoscope, cleanse and defog its tip, and reinsert it. By entering the abdomen superior to the site of hemorrhage, the bleeding vessel can usually be identified.

Because the moment of bleeding is unpredictable, the surgeon must be ready to respond to this problem when it occurs. The irrigator/aspirator must be on the field and operational at the *inception* of each laparoscopic procedure. This is the most valuable equipment for identifying and clearing the site of bleeding. The irrigant (1 L of saline with 5000 units of heparin added, with or without an antibiotic, e.g., 500 mg of cefazolin) must be pressurized to 250 mm Hg, and the suction tubing must be attached to the instrument and the suction should be operational. Alternatively, a gas-powered irrigation (700 mm Hg) suction unit can be used (e.g., Nezhat system).

In using electrosurgery to coagulate a blood vessel, the vessel will be sealed more effectively if the site of bleeding is occluded first with insulated grasping forceps. Electrocautery can then be applied to the jaws of the grasping forceps either directly, if the forceps can be connected to the electrosurgical unit, or indirectly by touching the jaws of the *insulated* closed forceps with the electrosurgical scissors. A *noninsulated* forceps should never be used for this purpose.

Alternatively, surgical clips can be applied. In this situation the surgeon will need to dissect the area on either side of the injured vessel to obtain a "window" around the entire circumference of the vessel so that the clips can be securely applied.

By first applying forceps to occlude the site of bleeding, the surgeon is certain that the site of bleeding has been identified before applying the coagulation current or a clip. "Blind" coagulation or "random" clipping usually will only make matters worse and may initiate a cascade culminating in emergency celiotomy.

Any vascular injury that results in hypotension or rapid accumulation of blood in the abdominal cavity requires an open surgical repair. A vascular surgeon should be consulted immediately. If emergency laparotomy becomes necessary, the laparoscopic sheath, if in a major vessel, should be left in place to tamponade the bleeding and guide the surgeon to the site of injury. Maintenance of the pneumoperitoneum allows for the rapid and safe entry into the peritoneal cavity, thereby reducing the risk of inadvertent injury to other abdominal structures. Once pressure control of the injured vessel has been achieved, the anesthesiologist should be given time to resuscitate the patient before initiating formal repair.

Alternatively, if the sheath has been removed from the vessel, it should be swung up toward the midline. The surgeon can then cut directly down onto the sheath, thereby rapidly entering the abdomen.

Perforation of a hollow viscus (bowel, bladder, stomach)

Problem During Veress needle or trocar insertion, the stomach, bowel, or bladder, may be entered.[37,39,44,45] Veress needle entry should be immediately apparent because of aspiration or irrigation/aspiration of gastrointestinal contents or of urine. Gastric dilation following mask ventilation, inadvertent esophageal intubation, or distended bowel increases the risk of gastrointestinal perforation.[45] If one of these conditions is suspected, an open approach should be considered, since the distended stomach or bowel will greatly increase the risk of a trocar injury. Similarly, a full bladder predisposes the patient to a bladder injury.

Rarely, patients with urachal abnormalities (i.e., cysts or sinuses) may be encountered. Because of its midline periumbilical location, a urachal abnormality places the patient at high risk for Veress needle or trocar perforation. A history of umbilical discharge should alert the surgeon to this possibility, and diagnostic studies should be performed before laparoscopy.[42,44]

Prevention For lengthier laparoscopic procedures or in high-risk patients (e.g., morbidly obese or markedly asthenic patients), a nasogastric or oral gastric tube should be placed after induction of anesthesia to ensure decompression of the stomach. Also, a proper bowel preparation will decompress the bowel and prepare it such that Veress needle perforation is both rare and inconsequential. Likewise, drainage of the bladder with a Foley catheter decreases the risk of bladder perforation.

Uncontrolled trocar introduction greatly increases the risk of injury to underlying intra-abdominal structures. Establishing an adequate pneumoperitoneum (i.e., intra-abdominal pressure can be momentarily raised to 25 mm Hg) before trocar insertion, incising the anterior abdominal wall fascia before trocar introduction, and the use of a braking technique that limits trocar excursion facilitate safe trocar placement.

Alternatively, if the patient is relatively thin, the surgeon may elect to keep the pneumoperitoneum pressure low (≤10 mm Hg) so he or she can firmly grasp and elevate the abdominal wall during initial trocar placement. Either method appears to work well. Once the initial port is placed, all subsequent trocar placements are performed during visual monitoring.

Because of the risk of adhesions, prior intra-abdominal surgery is a relative contraindication to the blind puncture technique for establishing the pneumoperitoneum. Depending on the nature of the prior procedure, it may be possible to introduce the Veress needle through a low-risk site (i.e., abdominal quadrant farthest away from the abdominal scar). Alternatively, these patients are ideal candidates for the minilaparotomy open (e.g., Hasson) cannula technique.

Unlike open surgical techniques, the laparoscopic surgeon is able to visualize only what is seen by the camera. Cutting and coagulating instruments outside the field of the camera can cause serious injury if not carefully observed. This is particularly true for unipolar electrosurgical instruments, which are commonly used. The use of shielded instruments, bipolar electrosurgery, and visualization of the *entire* "hot" (i.e., metallic) portion of the instrument when using the electrosurgery will decrease the risk of inadvertent injury to adjacent tissues.

In performing laparoscopy it is important to remember that the primary telescopic port was inserted blindly. Before beginning the procedure, the peritoneal point of entry of this trocar should be carefully inspected with a 5 or 10 mm laparoscope passed into one of the secondary ports; only in this manner can an inadvertent two-wall puncture of the bowel be noted early. Also, a full abdominal inspection should be done at the beginning and end of each laparoscopic procedure to rule out any visceral injury.

Diagnosis The passage of flatus or stool during the establishment of the initial pneumoperitoneum may indicate placement of the Veress needle within the bowel lumen. The presence of gas or blood in the urethral catheter drainage tubing or bag should alert the surgeon to a bladder injury. In this case intraoperative bladder distention with indigo-carmine–stained saline instilled via the urethral catheter may identify the cystotomy.

Treatment   Perforation of a hollow viscus with a Veress needle is of no consequence, whereas perforation of the same organ with a trocar must be repaired. For the skilled laparoscopist, this can be done using intracorporeal suturing or stapling techniques; under all other circumstances, an open repair is necessary. If unprepared bowel has been entered and there is significant fecal contamination, an open procedure is mandatory to obtain adequate exposure, effect a proper repair, and irrigate the abdomen; in this situation a diverting enterostomy may be necessary. If not already present, then consultation with a general surgeon is recommended.

Perforation of a solid viscus (liver, kidney, spleen)

Problem   Since the Veress needle and initial trocar are usually passed via a midline umbilical site, injury to a solid intra-abdominal organ is very unusual. Likewise, since all secondary trocars and instruments are passed under direct endoscopic control, solid organ injury should be rare.

Prevention   The Veress needle is introduced most safely at the umbilicus, thereby precluding injury to a solid organ. Furthermore, entry of all secondary trocars and auxiliary instrumentation is *always* endoscopically viewed, thereby decreasing the risk of solid organ injury.

Diagnosis   The problem of entry into a solid organ is noted at the time of Veress needle insertion: high CO_2 pressures, lack of CO_2 flow, and aspiration of blood or blood-tinged saline. Likewise, passage of a secondary trocar into a solid organ should be immediately apparent to the laparoscopist.

Treatment   The site of Veress needle injury of the liver or spleen can be directly electrocoagulated. Alternatively, the injury can be fulgurated with an argon beam coagulator, if available. Also, Avitene, oxycellulose sheets, or Gelfoam can be backloaded into the tip of a *dry* 5 or 10 mm suture introducer cannula. The tip of the cannula is placed directly over the site of injury, and the hemostatic agent is pushed out of the cannula directly and firmly onto the site of injury with a 5 or 10 mm blunt-tipped instrument, respectively.

If a significant trocar injury to a solid organ has occurred, open surgery will probably be necessary to repair the tear in the liver or to perform a splenectomy. If the kidney has sustained a trocar injury, the retroperitoneum will fill with blood and tamponade the site of injury. If the patient is otherwise stable, no further exploration is indicated. If the hematoma is expanding, open exploration is advised.

Peripheral nerve damage

Problem   Peripheral nerve damage in anesthetized patients is primarily the result of abnormal stretching or compression of a nerve. Of all the nerve groups, the brachial plexus is the most susceptible to nerve damage from malpositioning during anesthesia.[46] The use of shoulder braces with the patient in the head-down position pushes the clavicle into the retroclavicular space, which in turn exerts pressure on the brachial plexus.[47] Improper positioning of the patient's arms is another cause of brachial plexus injury, particularly if the arm is abducted beyond *90 degrees*. The head of the humerus can also exert excessive pressure on the brachial plexus if the arm is extremely rotated. Therefore the patients palms should be pronated (facing the thighs) to avoid external rotation of the humeral head when the arms are placed next to the trunk.[47] Femoral nerve damage during a diagnostic laparoscopy has been attributed to abduction and extreme lateral rotation of the hip joint in the dorsal lithotomy position.[48]

Prevention   As in all surgical procedures, careful attention to patient positioning and proper padding of bony prominences will decrease the risk of peripheral neuropathy. To avoid the use of shoulder braces, the patient can be secured to the operating room table at the level of the ankles, hips, and shoulders using Velcro straps or 3-inch strips of cloth tape. In addition, the arms should not be abducted >90 degrees. During laparoscopic procedures, the position of the operating room table may be changed many times. Each time the table is moved, the surgical team must be certain that the patient clears all of the surrounding structures, such as the nurse's Mayo stand and monitors, and be certain the patient is still properly padded.

Diagnosis   The diagnosis of a nerve palsy is made in the immediate postoperative period. For example, with a brachial plexus palsy, the patient, on awakening, will have significant loss of grip strength and will complain of numbness/tingling along the affected hand and lower arm.

Treatment   Once a peripheral nerve injury has occurred, little can be done to reverse the damage. Nerve conduction studies can be performed to document acute denervation and establish a baseline for future comparison. Physical therapy should also be instituted to avoid atrophy of the muscles innervated by the damaged nerve. Mild palsies usually resolve in 4 to 6 weeks. Following severe stretch injury or cutting of a nerve, recovery may take as long as 2 years, if it occurs at all.

POSTOPERATIVE COMPLICATIONS

Fever/peritonitis

Problem   The postoperative occurrence of fever and abdominal wall tenderness (i.e., rebound) may be the first sign of a "missed" intra-operative bowel perforation.[49]

Prevention   Bowel injury results from blind passage of instruments or trocars into the abdomen or from use of an electrosurgical probe when the entire "live" metal portion is not in the field of view.

Diagnosis   The diagnosis can be suggested from clinical signs and an obstructive series. If there is still doubt as to the diagnosis, a CT scan of the abdomen with oral contrast can be obtained; this may show oral contrast lying outside of the alimentary tract.

Treatment   Surgical exploration, peritoneal lavage, and a diverting enterostomy constitute the recommended course of action.

Delayed hemorrhage

Problem   The differential diagnosis for postoperative hemodynamic instability includes a number of possible causes: myocardial infarction, pulmonary embolus, sepsis, hypervolemia or hypovolemia, and acute blood loss. Although diagnosis of each of these is of critical importance, ongoing blood loss is the problem most directly attributable to the laparoscopic procedure.

Prevention   Establishing hemostasis before the completion of a procedure is a requirement of all laparoscopic interventions; active bleeding should not be expected to disappear once the monitoring camera is removed. At the end of each procedure, the pneumoperitoneum is decreased to 5 mm Hg and a thorough abdominal inspection for bleeding is completed. Also, the anterior abdominal wall at the sites of trocar insertion is a commonly overlooked cause of delayed hemorrhage. This is particularly true at the lateral trocar insertion sites in the region of the inferior epigastric vessels. Again, the peritoneal side of *all* trocar insertion sites should be visualized at the end of the procedure at 5 mm Hg to exclude them as potential sites of active bleeding.

Diagnosis   Prolonged (i.e., >24 hours) or newly developing post-operative pain, abdominal distention, and a slowly falling hematocrit are all symptoms and signs of a delayed hemorrhage.

Treatment   The management of postoperative bleeding is dependent on the hemodynamic significance of this problem and as such varies from immediate open surgical exploration to observation. If the latter option is selected, a CT scan of the abdomen and possibly a chromium-labeled red blood cell study may be indicated to identify the size of the hematoma and the presence or absence of significant ongoing bleeding, respectively.

Incisional hernia

Problem   The risk of herniation of abdominal contents through the trocar insertion sites depends on the trocar size. The ≤5 mm trocar sites are at low risk for the late development of incisional hernias, whereas herniation may occur via the ≥10 mm peritoneotomies.

Prevention   For trocar insertion sites ≥10 mm, the fascia is approximated with a single figure-of-eight absorbable suture (e.g., 0 absorbable suture on a TT-3 needle). This is done with the abdomen still insufflated and under laparoscopic monitoring via a 5 mm laparoscope passed through a 5 mm port; this precludes inadvertent injury to the underlying abdominal viscera.

Diagnosis   Development of localized abdominal discomfort several days after the procedure is a symptom of a herniation through one of the ≥10 mm port sites. Physical examination may reveal a palpable bulge at the previous port site. The mass itself may be tender or non-tender, depending on the degree of entrapment of the bowel or omentum.

Treatment   The laparoscopic incisional hernia can be reduced via a second laparoscopic procedure. The fascial site can then be closed with intracorporeal laparoscopic or standard open suturing techniques.

Azotemia

Problem   Azotemia, especially if associated with ascites and hyponatremia, may be secondary to an unrecognized intraoperative bladder perforation. A cystogram will confirm the diagnosis; flexible cystoscopy will accurately determine the location and size of the injury. Macroscopic hematuria or pneumaturia in the recovery room is indicative of a possible unrecognized cystotomy.

Prevention   There are two ways in which vesical trauma can be minimized: bladder decompression with a Foley urethral catheter and taking care during all pelvic procedures to identify and *if possible* to remain lateral to the medial umbilical ligament. Also, the blind insertion of trocars or instruments should always be avoided.

Diagnosis   A rising serum creatinine level associated with hyperkalemia and hyponatremia is indicative of an "unrecognized" bladder perforation. Typically, there is slight abdominal distention, although the abdomen remains nontender. The urine initially is blood tinged; however, by the first postoperative day, there may be no macroscopic hematuria and only scant microhematuria.

Treatment If the cystotomy is small (<5 mm), it should resolve with 2 weeks of continuous bladder catheter drainage. However, if the cystotomy is large, then open or possibly laparoscopic repair is indicated.

CONCLUSION

In laparoscopy, as in all areas of surgery, experience, knowledge, and meticulous attention to detail are the most important factors in avoiding complications. In this regard prevention is always preferable to treatment (see box on p. 217); however, when problems arise, knowledgeable and expeditious treatment becomes essential to successfully salvage the laparoscopic procedure.

REFERENCES

1. Winfield HN, Donovan JF, See WA, Loening SA, Williams RD. Urological laparoscopic surgery. J Urol 146:941-948, 1991.
2. Mintz M. Risks and prophylaxis in laparoscopy: A survey of 100,000 cases. J Reprod Med 18:269-272, 1977.
3. Fishburne JI, Keith L. Anesthesia. In Laparoscopy. Baltimore: Williams & Wilkins, 1977, pp 69-85.
4. Scott DB, Julian DG. Observations on cardiac arrhythmias during laparoscopy. Br Med J 1:411-413, 1972.
5. Graff TD, Arbegast NR, Phillips OC, Harris LC, Frazer TM. Gas embolism: A comparative study of air and carbon dioxide as embolic agents in the systemic venous system. Am J Obstet Gynecol 78:259-265, 1959.
6. Östman PL, Pantle-Fisher FH, Faure EA, Glosten B. Circulatory collapse during laparoscopy. J Clin Anesth 2:129-132, 1990.
7. Brantley JC, Riley PM. Cardiovascular collapse during laparoscopy: A report of two cases. Am J Obstet Gynecol 159:735-737, 1988.
8. Clark CC, Weeks DB, Gusdon JP. Venous carbon dioxide embolism during laparoscopy. Anesth Analg 56:650-652, 1977.
9. Bradfield ST. Gas embolism during laparoscopy. Anaesth Intensive Care 19:474, 1991.
10. De Plater RMH, Jones ISC. Non-fatal carbon dioxide embolism during laparoscopy. Anaesth Intensive Care 17:359-361, 1989.
11. Root B, Levy MN, Pollack SW, Lubert M, Pathak K. Gas embolism death after laparoscopy delayed by "trapping" in portal circulation. Anesth Analg 57:232-237, 1978.
12. Yacoub OF, Cardona I, Coveler LA, Dodson MG. Carbon dioxide embolism during laparoscopy. Anesthesiology 57:533-535, 1982.
13. Bedford RF. Venous air embolism: A historical perspective. Semin Anesth 2:169-176, 1983.
14. Shapiro HM, Drummond JC. Neurosurgical anesthesia and intracranial hypertension. In Anesthesia. New York: Churchill Livingstone, 1990, pp 1737-1789.

15. Lenz RJ, Thomas TA, Wilkins DG. Cardiovascular changes during laparoscopy. Anaesthesia 31:4-12, 1976.
16. Kashtan J, Green JF, Parsons EQ, Holcroft JW. Hemodynamic effects of increased abdominal pressure. J Surg Res 30:249-255, 1981.
17. Kelman GR, Swapp GH, Smith I, Benzie RJ, Gordon NLM. Cardiac output and arterial blood-gas tension during laparoscopy. Br J Anaesth 44:1155-1161, 1972.
18. Motew M, Ivankovich AD, Bieniarz J, et al. Cardiovascular effects and acid-base and blood gas changes during laparoscopy. Am J Obstet Gynecol 115:1002-1011, 1973.
19. Johannsen G, Andersen M, Juhl B. The effect of general anesthesia on the hemodynamic events during laparoscopy with CO_2-insufflation. Acta Anaesthesiol Scand 33:132-136, 1989.
20. Bedford RF, Feinstein B. Hospital admission blood pressure: A prediction for hypertension following endotracheal intubation. Anesth Analg 59:367-370, 1980.
21. Harris MNE, Plantevin OM, Crowther A. Cardiac arrhythmias during anesthesia for laparoscopy. Br J Anaesth 56:1213-1217, 1984.
22. Scott DB. Some effects of peritoneal insufflation of carbon dioxide at laparoscopy. Anaesthesia 25:590, 1970.
23. Myles PS. Arrhythmias during laparoscopy. Br J Anaesth 63:365, 1989.
24. Doyle DJ, Mark PWS. Laparoscopy and vagal arrest. Anaesthesia 44:448, 1989.
25. Katz RL, Bigger JT. Cardiac arrhythmias during anesthesia and operation. Anesthesiology 33:193-213, 1970.
26. Inglis JM, Brooke BN. Trendelenburg tilt—an obsolete position. Br Med J 2:343-344, 1956.
27. Altschule MD. The significance of changes in the lung volume and its subdivisions during and after abdominal operations. Anesthesiology 4:385-391, 1943.
28. Wilcox S, Vandam LD. Alas, poor Trendelenburg and his position. Anesth Analg 67:574-578, 1988.
29. Carmichael DE. Laparoscopy—cardiac consideration. Fertil Steril 22:69-70, 1971.
30. Hodgson C, McClelland RMA, Newton JR. Some effect of the peritoneal insufflation of carbon dioxide at laparoscopy. Anaesthesia 25:382-390, 1970.
31. Alexander GD, Noe FE, Brown EM. Anesthesia for pelvic laparoscopy. Anesth Analg 48:14-18, 1969.
32. Ciofolo MJ, Clergue F, Seebacher J, Lefebvre G, Viars P. Ventilatory effects of laparoscopy under epidural anesthesia. Anesth Analg 70:357-361, 1990.
33. Brown DR, Fishburne JI, Roberson VO, Hulka JF. Ventilatory and blood gas changes during laparoscopy with local anesthesia. Am J Obstet Gynecol 124:741-745, 1976.
34. Duffy BL. Regurgitation during pelvic laparoscopy. Br J Anaesth 51:1089-1090, 1979.
35. Carlsson C, Islander G. Silent gastropharyngeal regurgitation during anesthesia. Anesth Analg 60:655-657, 1981.
36. Kurer FL, Welch DB. Gynaecological laparoscopy: Clinical experiences of two anaesthetic techniques. Br J Anaesth 56:1207-1211, 1984.
37. Saleh JW. Complications. In Laparoscopy. Philadelphia: WB Saunders, 1988, pp 253-266.
38. Kalhan SB, Reaney JA, Collins RL. Pneumomediastinum and subcutaneous emphysema during laparoscopy. Cleve Clin J Med 47:639-642, 1990.
39. Pascual JB, Baranda MM, Tarrero MT, Gutierrez MFM, Garrido IM, Errasti CA. Subcutaneous emphysema, pneumomediastinum, bilateral pneumothorax, and pneumopericardium after laparoscopy. Endoscopy 22:59, 1990.
40. Doctor NH, Hussain Z. Bilateral pneumothorax associated with laparoscopy. Anaesthesia 28:75-81, 1973.

41. Altman AR, Johnson TH. Pneumoperitoneum and pneumoretroperitoneum. Consequences of positive end-expiratory pressure therapy. Arch Surg 114:208-211, 1979.
42. Yuzpe AA. Pneumoperitoneum needle and trocar injuries in laparoscopy. J Reprod Med 35:484-490, 1990.
43. Pierson DJ. Chest tubes. In Critical Care Medicine. Philadelphia: WB Saunders, 1988, pp 238-246.
44. Penfield AJ. Trocar and needle injuries. In Laparoscopy. Baltimore: Williams & Wilkins, 1977, pp 236-241.
45. Reynolds RC, Pauca AL. Gastric perforation, an anesthesia-induced hazard in laparoscopy. Anesthesiology 38:84-85, 1973.
46. Britt BA, Joy N, Makay MB. Positioning trauma. In Complications in Anesthesiology. Philadelphia: JB Lippincott, 1983, pp 646-670.
47. Prentice JA, Martin JT. The Trendelenburg position—anesthesiologic considerations. In Positioning in Anesthesia and Surgery. Philadelphia: WB Saunders, 1987, pp 127-145.
48. Hershlag A, Loy RA, Lavy G, De Cherney AH. Femoral neuropathy after laparoscopy. J Reprod Med 35:575-576, 1990.
49. Yong EL, Prabhakaran K, Lee YS, Ratnan SS. Peritonitis following diagnostic laparoscopy due to injury to a vesicourachal diverticulum. Case report. Br J Obstet Gynaecol 96:365-368, 1989.
50. Shifren JL, Adelstein L, Finkler NJ. Asystolic cardiac arrest: A rare complication of laparoscopy. Obstet Gynecol 79:840-841, 1992.

CHAPTER 14

Pediatric Applications of Laparoscopy

Louis R. Kavoussi, Diane F. Merritt, and Randall R. Odem

The pioneers of endoscopy in children were Stephen Gans and George Berci. They reported performing laparoscopy in newborns weighing as little as 1800 g and as young as 1 day of age.[1] While the use of laparoscopy is widespread in most surgical disciplines, this approach has only recently gained acceptance for use in children. The indications for laparoscopy in children and its specific points merit special discussion.

SPECIAL CONSIDERATIONS IN PEDIATRIC LAPAROSCOPY

Several considerations are important in pediatric laparoscopy. First, as in the thin patient, there is a relatively short distance between the anterior abdominal wall and the great vessels; thus trocars and needles must not be passed too deeply to avoid vascular injuries. Also, the abdominal fascia is thinner in the child, so less pressure is needed to introduce the Veress needle or trocars into the abdomen (Fig. 14-1).

A small child's liver is proportionally larger and in infants is palpable 1 to 2 cm below the right costal margin. A spleen tip may be palpated

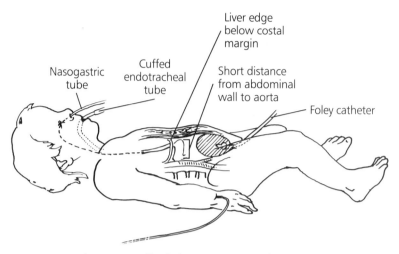

Fig. 14-1 Pediatric laparoscopy: patient set-up.

in normal infants at the left costal margin. The stomach lies in a horizontal position in infancy, accounting for increased postprandial abdominal protuberance in the epigastric area. The more vertical adult position of the stomach develops gradually throughout childhood.[2]

Pelvic anatomy differs in infants and young children. A large portion of the bladder is located outside the bony pelvis; therefore decompression of the bladder with a catheter before Veress needle or trocar introduction is essential to avoid a bladder perforation. The child's peritoneal cavity is small compared with that of adults; thus much less total gas, as little as 300 cc, is required to achieve an adequate pneumoperitoneum (see Fig. 14-1).

ANESTHESIA

General endotracheal anesthesia with a cuffed tube, pluse oximetry, and end-tidal CO_2 monitoring are used in pediatric laparoscopy. The child must not move during the procedure. The child's respirations are very sensitive to the insufflation pressure; thus mechanical ventilation is usually required, and intra-abdominal pressure is maintained at ≤10 to 15 mm Hg. Also, during prolonged procedures children can absorb a significant amount of CO_2 and thus are at an increased risk for the development of hypercarbia.

PATIENT PREPARATION

Before Veress needle placement, the bladder needs to be drained with a urethral catheter. A nasogastric or an orogastric tube should be placed to decompress the stomach. A preoperative bowel preparation is not needed.

VERESS NEEDLE PLACEMENT

When placing the Veress needle, a right-handed physician should stand on the patient's left side and vice versa. The patient should be in a 30-degree head-down position to help displace the intestines from the pelvis. The needle should be grasped close to its tip to avoid penetrating the abdomen too deeply. The needle is inserted through a small incision at the base of the umbilicus. A towel clip may be used to grasp the lower lip of the umbilicus and raise it slightly anteriorly as the needle is passed. The tip of the needle is aimed toward the pelvis (30 degrees). Tests for determining proper needle placement are as described for the adult patient (see Chapter 4).

INSUFFLATION

Insufflation should progress at a rate of ≤ 1 L/min, since a relatively small volume of CO_2 may be sufficient to obtain a pneumoperitoneum; in some instances as little as 300 cc is all that is needed. The intra-abdominal pressure should be watched carefully because small increments in gas introduced into the peritoneum can result in marked elevations in intra-abdominal pressure; the insufflation pressure should always be kept below 15 mm Hg. Higher pressure, especially in infants, can lead to difficulties with ventilation, impaired venous return, and hypercarbia.

TROCAR PLACEMENT

When placing trocars, it is again important not to advance ports too deeply to avoid injury to underlying bowel or vascular structures. Fixing and raising the abdomen 1 cm anteriorly with towel clips at the planned site of port placement may be helpful. In neonates and young infants, the umbilical fascia may be quite thin and leakage of gas may occur around a trocar placed in this location. Thus, *to avoid loss of pneumoperitoneum, the trocar can be placed just inferior to the umbilicus.*

Once the initial 10 or 5 mm camera trocar is in position, the abdomen is inspected with either the 10 or 5 mm laparoscope to rule out any injury that may have occurred during Veress needle or trocar placement.

All other ports are placed under direct vision. The light of the laparo-scope is used to transilluminate the abdominal wall at potential trocar sites to detect and thus avoid injuring any underlying abdominal wall vessels while passing the secondary trocars.

INSTRUMENTATION

Standard laparoscopy sets contain 5 mm sheaths and a 5 mm laparo-scope. This equipment, although a bit on the long side, is adequate in most instances of diagnostic pediatric laparoscopy.

The shorter pediatric instruments, however, are obviously easier to use. The trocars range from 3 to 6 mm in diameter, and their lengths vary from 15 to 20 cm. Shorter grasping instruments are easier to ma-nipulate than their longer adult counterparts. A 5 mm laparoscope with a 6 Fr working channel is available, although the optical resolution and image clarity are not as good as with the 10 mm laparoscope.

APPLICATIONS

Laparoscopy has been used in the pediatric population for more than 20 years, primarily as a diagnostic procedure for exploration of various pathologic states of the internal reproductive organs, evaluation of chronic pelvic pain, and evaluation of cholestasis and liver disease. Laparoscopy in children has been used to direct liver biopsies and in the differential diagnosis of biliary atresia and choledochal cysts.[1,3]

Under most circumstances laparoscopy is used in children to avoid laparotomy. In some cases laparoscopy may provide definitive infor-mation that leads to the necessity of performing a laparotomy.[4] Lapa-roscopy permits thorough inspection of the uterus, tubes, ovaries, blad-der, gallbladder, cecum, appendix, and spleen. Partial evaluation of the liver, colon, distal ureter, pelvic lymph nodes, undersurface of the di-aphragm, small intestine, and stomach may be readily accomplished by laparoscopy.

There is limited ability to assess retroperitoneal structures; however, laparoscopic nephrectomy has been successfully reported in a 6-month-old infant and in two adolescents. Laparoscopic ureterolysis has been successfully accomplished in a 15-year-old girl for idiopathic retroper-itoneal fibrosis. In the future laparoscopy may have a role in staging pediatric patients with urologic malignancies (i.e., Wilms' tumor, neu-roblastoma, rhabdomyosarcoma) or in treating asymptomatic vari-oceles. As surgeons' skills and familiarity with laparoscopic procedures improve, reconstructive procedures such as ureteral reimplantation and pyeloplasty may be performed laparoscopically.[5] The gonadal applications of pediatric laparoscopy include diagnostic evaluation of the cryptorchid or intersex patient, orchiectomy for a dysplastic intra-abdominal testicle or gonadectomy in a patient with intersex, and the first stage of a Fowler-Stephens maneuver.[5] An important use is in determining the nature of pelvic organs in intersex or gonadal problems.

Gynecologic literature from the 1960s and 1970s described liberal use of the laparoscope for the diagnosis of primary and secondary amenorrhea.[6] Currently, noninvasive state-of-the-art cytogenetic, hormonal, and sonographic studies obviate the need for performing diagnostic laparoscopy to confirm such diagnoses as müllerian agenesis, polycystic ovaries, gonadal dysgenesis, and precocious puberty. An exception might be in the case in which documentation of 45,X/46,XX, or 45,X, 46,XY mosaicism by ovarian biopsy may be of value in the management of such patients. The prompt use of diagnostic laparoscopy in the evaluation of adnexal torsion in children will result in an increased salvage rate of torsed adnexa and has great advantage over "expectant" management in questionable cases of abdominal pain. In childhood, adnexal torsion may involve normal tissue. In this young population, preservation of reproductive potential is of utmost importance, and conservative management is indicated. Reduction of a forced adnexal structure can easily be accomplished by laparoscopy if the structure involved appears ischemic and not yet gangrenous.[7,8]

A laparoscopic splenectomy was performed for a girl with autoimmune thrombocytopenic purpura.[9]

Cholelithiasis is not a common condition in childhood, but does occur in patients with hemolytic disease, such as sickle cell disease, thalassemia, and hereditary spherocytosis. Less commonly recognized pathologic factors for cholelithiasis in children include long-term parenteral nutrition, ileum disease or resection, history of severe infection or volume depletion, cystic fibrosis, and anatomic abnormalities of the biliary tract.[2] Laparoscopic cholecystectomy has been described by several authors in 18 children, ranging in age from 19 months to 17 years.[2,10-12]

Alain et al.[13] reported performing extramucosal pylorotomy by laparoscopy in 10 children with congenital hypertrophic pyloric stenosis. The laparoscopic approach to Nissen fundoplication is relatively new, yet it has been reported for the treatment of gastroesophageal reflux in a 10-year-old boy.[14]

Gotz et al.[15] reported the results of 388 laparoscopic appendectomies (40% pediatric). Valla et al.[16] reported a large series of 465 cases of laparoscopic appendectomy in children, who ranged in age from 3 to 16 years.

While the primary diagnosis of intra-abdominal tumors is possible through laparoscopy, its use as a "second look" procedure for possible recurrent malignancy or for staging in Hodgkins disease is of value. Laparoscopy for the diagnosis of intra-abdominal trauma has been reported.[4] Other potenital uses of laparoscopy include retrieval of ventriculoperitoneal shunt catheters. Entrapment, displacement, or cyst formation can be diagnosed and corrected endoscopically.[17] Before radiation therapy, the ovarian pedicles of a 7-year-old child were marked by laparoscopically placed steel clips to limit irradiation to the gonads during treatment of a sacral tumor.

Laparoscopy has been used for the diagnosis and treatment of abdominal pain in adolescent girls. Several series of pediatric and adolescent cases have been reported by Gans and Berci,[1] Leape and Ramenofsky,[4] Kleinhaus et al.,[18] Goldstein et al.,[19] Cognat et al.,[6] and Wolfman and Kreutner.[20] In this population the laparoscopic findings include endometriosis, postoperative adhesions, uterine anomalies, pelvic inflammatory disease, functional ovarian cysts, paraovarian cysts, and adnexal torsion. Postoperatively a videotape of the laparoscopic findings may be reviewed with the patient and family as part of the treatment process. Even when no pathologic condition is seen in these pateints, there is a great therapeutic advantage, so that psychosocial support for these patients may then proceed with confidence.

With the applications of operative laparoscopy developing so rapidly, it is likely that newer techniques will be added faster than publications or controlled studies can be generated. Although endoscopic approaches offer practical alternatives—such as decreased morbidity and shorter hospital stays compared with conventional surgery—for some patients and some disorders, conventional open operative procedures will remain the wiser choice. Just because something is new does not mean it is better.[17] Before laparoscopic procedures become widely adopted in pediatric surgery, careful attention will have to be paid to the appropriate training of surgeons.

TROUBLESHOOTING

All laparoscopic problems that can occur during adult laparoscopy can also occur in children. However, the following problems are unique to the child or to the previously discussed surgical procedures.

Problem: Asthenic child: short distance between the abdominal wall and the underlying viscera.

Solution: During the passage of Veress needle, primary trocars, and secondary trocars, towel clips can be used on either side of the needle/

trocars to slightly elevate and stabilize the abdominal wall away from the abdominal contents. Alternatively, the surgeon can use his or her nondominant hand to grasp the lower midline of the abdomen and hold it upward.

Problem: Omental evisceration has been described through small (5 mm) laparoscopic ports following laparoscopy in young children. This problem may be peculiar to asthenic children and adults in whom the omentum is thin and membrane like.[21]
Solution: Omental evisceration is possible through small laparoscopic puncture sites in spite of fascial closure. Additional measures to prevent omental evisceration include: removal of instruments in descending order of port size and under endoscopic monitoring, elevation of the abdominal wall with the removal of the final sheath, and closure of each fascial defect under direct vision with absorbable sutures and use of the sutures to elevate the anterior fascia during tying to avoid entrapment of omentum or viscera.[21]

Problem: In the asthenic child dislodgement of the trocar sleeve and loss of pneumoperitoneum can occur.
Solution: Use of surgigrips on the sleeves. Avoid making too large of an incision for the trocar. Placement of the trocar slightly lateral to umbilicus, through the rectus muscle, avoids the periumbilical area.

REFERENCES

1. Gans SL, Berci G. Peritoneoscopy in infants and children. J Pediatr Surg 8:399, 1973.
2. Rosser JC, Boeckman CR, Andrews D. Laparoscopic cholecystectomy in an infant. Surg Laparosc Endosc 2:143, 1992.
3. Gans SL, Berci G. Advances in endoscopy of infants and children. J Pediatr Surg 6:199, 1971.
4. Leape LL, Ramenofsky ML. Laparoscopy in children. Pediatrics 66:215, 1980.
5. Kavoussi LR. Pediatric applications of laparoscopy. In Clayman RV, McDougall EM (eds). Laparoscopic Urology. St. Louis: Quality Medical Publishing, 1993, p 209.
6. Cognat M, Rosenberg D, David L, Papathanassiou Z. Laparoscopy in infants and adolescents. Obstet Gynecol 42:515, 1973.
7. Merritt DF. Torsion of the uterine adnexa: A review. Adolesc Pediatr Gynecol 4:3, 1991.
8. Shalev E, Mann S, Romano S, Rahav D. Laparoscopic detorsion of adnexa in childhood: A case report. J Pediatr Surg 26:1193, 1991.
9. Delaitre B, Maignien B. Laparoscopic splenectomy—technical aspects. Surg Endosc 6:305, 1992.
10. Holcomb GW III, Olsen DO, Sharp KW. Laparoscopic cholecystectomy in the pediatric patient. J Pediatr Surg 26:1186, 1991.
11. Newman KD, Marmon LM, Attori R, Evens S. Laparoscopic cholecystectomy in pediatric patients. J Pediatr Surg 26:1184, 1991.

12. Moir CR, Donohue JH, van Heerden JA. Laparoscopic cholecystectomy in children: Initial experience and recommendations. J Pediatr Surg 27:1066, 1992.
13. Alain JL, Grousseau D, Terrier G. Extramucosal pylorotomy by laparoscopy. J Pediatr Surg 26:1191, 1991.
14. Lobe TE, Schropp KP, Lunsford K. Laparoscopic Nissen fundoplication in childhood. J Pediatr Surg 28:358, 1993.
15. Gotz F, Pier A, Bacher C. Modified laparoscopic appendectomy in surgery. Surg Endosc 4:6, 1990.
16. Valla JS, Limonne B, Valla V, Montupet P, Daoud N, Grinda A, Chavrier Y. Laparoscopic appendectomy in children: Report of 465 cases. Surg Laparosc Endosc 1:166, 1991.
17. Bloom DA, Ritchey ML, Jordon GH. Pediatric peritoneoscopy (laparoscopy). Clin Pediatr 5:100, 1993.
18. Kleinhaus S, Hein K, Sheran M, Boley S. Laparoscopy for diagnosis and treatment of abdominal pain in adolescent girls. Arch Surg 112:1178, 1977.
19. Goldstein DP, deCholnoky C, Emans SJ, Leventhal JM. Laparoscopy in the diagnosis and management of pelvic pain in adolescents. J Reprod Med 24:251, 1980.
20. Wolfman WL, Kreutner K. Laparoscopy in children and adolescents. J Adolesc Health Care 5:261, 1984.
21. Bloom DA, Ehrlich RM. Omental evisceration through small laparoscopy port sites. J Endourol 7:31, 1993.
22. Gundy JH. The pediatric physical exam. In Hoekelman RA, Friedman SB, Nelson NM, Seidel HM (eds). Primary Pediatric Care (2nd ed). St. Louis: Mosby–Year Book, 1992.

APPENDICES

Instrumentation

Paramjit S. Chandhoke

Table A-1 Pneumoperitoneum

Instrument	Features	Advanced Surgical	Cabot Medical	Circon ACMI	Dexide	Elmed	Ethicon Endo-Surgery	Jarit
Veress needle		12,15 cm	10,14 cm	X	12,15 cm	10,13,15 cm	X	12,15 cm
CO_2 insufflator	Low flow, 1-4 L/min					X		
	High flow, up to 6-10 L/min		+N_2O yoke	X		X		
	Automatic, 1 or 7 L/min							

			Manufacturers					
Marlow Surgical	Nortech	Olympus	Origin Medsystems	Storz	U.S. Surgical	Linvatec	Haraeus Surgical	Wolf
X	X	X	12,15 cm	X	12,15 cm	X	X	X
				X			X	X
X	+N$_2$O yoke, with recir- culation			10 L/min 20 L/min			X	X
							X	X

Table A-2 Trocars

	Manufacturers							
Diameter	Cabot Medical	Circon ACMI	Cook Urological	Dexide	Elmed	Ethicon Endo-Surgery	Jarit	Ma Su
3 mm					P, C, SV, ND, RS			
5 mm	P, C, TV, D, ND			D, GV, RS, SRS, SS, SV	P, C, SV, ND, RS	P, GV, D, SRS, SS	CV, P, SV, ND, RS, SRS	P, T D
5.5 mm	P, C, TV, ND	P, TV, ND, RS		D, GV, RS, SRS, SS, SV				
5.8/6.0 mm					P, C, TV, ND, RS			
7 mm	P, TV, D					P, GV, D, SRS, SS		
8 mm	P, TV, ND, D				P, C, TV, ND, RS			
10 mm	P, C, TV, D, ND		L = 150; P, SV, ND	D, GV, RS, SRS, SS, SV	P, C, TV, ND, RS	P, GV, D, SRS, SS	CV, P, TV, ND, RS	P, T D
11 mm	P, C, TV, D, ND	P, TV, ND, RS		D, GV, RS, SRS, SS, SV	P, C, TV, ND, RS	P, GV, D, SRS, SS	CV, P, TV, ND, RS	P, T R
12 mm	P, TV, ND, D		L = 150; P, SV, ND	D, GV, RS, SRS, SS, SV		P, GV, D, SRS, SS	CV, P, RS, SRS, TV	P, T R
15 mm	P, TV, ND		L = 150; P, SV, ND					
18 mm						X		
22 mm								
33 mm						X		

*Trocar length in centimeters.
ABBREVIATIONS: C = conical tip; CV = clip valve; D = disposable; DR = dilation rod; GV = gasket valve; L = length in millimete
ND = nondisposable; P = pyramidal tip; R = reducers in 3.5, 4.5, 5.0, 5.5, 7.5, and 10.5 mm sizes; RS = reducer sleeves: 11-5
8-7 mm, 8-5 mm, 7-5 mm, 5-4 mm; SRS = self-retaining sleeve; SS = safety shield; SV = septa silicone valve; TV = trumpet v

			Manufacturers				
Nortech	Olympus	Origin Medsystems	Storz*	U.S. Surgical	Linvatec	Haraeus Surgical	Wolf
				L = 70; P, D, SS			P, C, CV, ND
P, TV, ND	P, TV, ND, RS	L = 70, 100; P, D, R	L = 10.5; C, P, TV, ND, RS	L = 70, 100; P, D, SS	P, TV, ND		P, C, CV, DR, ND, SS
			L = 10.5; C, P, TV, ND, RS			L = 95, 125; P, C, TV, DR, ND	
			L = 10.5; C, P, TV, ND, R			L = 95, 125; P, C, TV, DR, ND	
			L = 10.5; C, P, TV, ND, RS	L = 100; P, D, SS			P, C, TV, ND
				L = 100; P, D, SS			P, TV, ND, RS
	P, TV, ND, RS	L = 100; P, D, R	L = 10.5; C, P, TV, ND, RS	L = 100, 150; P, D, SS	P, TV, ND	Hasson trocar	P, C, TV, ND
P, TV, ND, RS	P, TV, ND, RS, DR	L = 100; P, D, R	L = 10.5; C, P, TV, ND, R	L = 100; P, D, SS	P, TV, ND, Hasson trocar	L = 95, 125; P, C, TV, ND	
		L = 100; P, D, R	L = 11.5; C, P, TV, ND, RS	L = 70, 100, 150; P, D, SS			P, C, TV, ND
			L = 12; P, ND, RS	L = 100; P, D, SS		L = 95, 125; P, C, TV, ND	
			X				

Table A-3 Endoscopic equipment

Instrument	Features	Cabot Medical	Circon ACMI	Dexide	Elmed	Jarit	Marlow Surgical	Medical Dynamics
					Manufacturers			
Endoscopes	1.7 mm							
	2.7/4.0 mm		0°, 30°		30°			Optical catheter
	5 mm	0°	0°		0°, OS	0°, 30°	0°, 30°	0°
	6.5/7.0 mm				0°, OS			
	8 mm	0°						
	10 mm	0°, 30°	0°, 30°		0°, OS	0°, 30°, OS	0°, OS	0°
	11/12 mm				0°, OS			
Antifog solution				FRED	X			
Light source		HI, FO, MH, Xe	MH, Xe		HI, FO			MH, Xe
Camera		X	DC, BS		X			X
Video monitor	13 in	HR	HR, UHR		X			HR
tor	19/20 in	HR	HR, UHR					HR
Monitor cart		X	X		X			X
Video recorder		½ in, ¾ in	½ in, ¾ in, beta, 8 mm					X
Audio recording			X					
Video printer		X	X					X

ABBREVIATIONS: BS = beam splitter; DC = direct coupler; FO = fiberoptic; HI = high intensity; HR = high resolution; LO = low intensity; MH = metal halide; OC = operating channel; OS = offset lens; UHR = ultra high resolution; Xe = xenon.

				Manufacturers				
Merocel	MP Video	Nortech	Olympus	Origin Medsystems	Storz	Linvatec	Haraeus Surgical	Wolf
				0° FO				
					0°, 6°, 30°, 70°, 120°			5°, 70°
		0°	5°		0°, 30°	0°	0°, 30°	0°, 25°, 50°
					0°, 30°		30°	0°, 25°, 50°, 3 mm OC
					0°, 30°			
		0°	0°		0°, 30°, 45°, 0° = OL, OC	0°	0°, 30°	0°, 25°, 50°, 3 mm OC
					0°, 6°, OL, OC		0°, 30°, 6 mm OC	10°, 8 mm OC
ELVIS					U.F.O.	Ultra-stop		
	MH, HI		Xe	HI, Xe	Xe	MH, Xe	HI	HI/LO
	X		X	UHR	X	DC, BS	DC, BS	DC, BS
	HR		HR, UHR		HR	HR		HR
	HR		HR		HR	HR		HR
	X		X		X	X		X
	X		½ in		½ in, ¾ in	½ in, ¾ in, 8 mm		½ in
	X		X		X	X		X

Table A-4 — Grasping, holding, cutting, coagulation, and retraction*

	Manufacturers						
Instrument	Advanced Surgical	Cabot Medical	Circon ACMI	Cook Urological	Elmed	Ethicon Endo-Surgery	Jarit
Allis tooth grasper	E		X		X	E, D	I, N, RT
Alligator forceps			X	X	X	E, D	I, U
Angled dissecting forceps			X		X		I, U, NI, 5, 10 mm
Babcock forceps			X		X	E, D	NI, RT, 5, 10 mm
Biopsy forceps	I, WT		X	NI	3, 5, 11 mm, E		I, U, NI, WT
Biopsy punch	I				X		I, U, WT
Bowel grasper	NI	NI			X	E, D	NI
Claw forceps	NI, 11 mm	NI, 5, 11 mm			11 mm, E		NI, 5, 10 mm
Coagulating dissecting forceps, U	E					E, D	I, U, 5, 10 mm
Coagulating forceps, B	E	E			3, 5 mm, E		E
Coagulating electrode	E, WS	E			3, 5 mm, E	E, D	E, WS, I
Cobra-toothed grasper	I, RT				X		
Curved dissecting forceps			E, I		X	E, D	I, E, U, 5, 10 mm
Curved scissors			E, I		3, 5 mm, E	E, D	E, U, I
Dissecting forceps	NI		E, I			E, D	E, U, I, 5, 10 mm
Dissecting hook			E, I		X	E, D	NI, I, E, 5, 10 mm
Duck-bill grasper	I, RT		E, I				RT
Endocoagulator	E				E		
Grasping forceps, A	I, NI		E, I		3, 5 mm, E	E, D	I, NI, RT, 5, 10 mm
Grasping forceps, T	E, NI, RT		E, I		3, 5, 11 mm, E	E, D	RT, I, NI, 5, 10 mm
Hasson graspers			NI				
Hook electrode	E		E, I	E	3, 5 mm, E		E, WS, I
Hook scissors	I		E, I			E, D	E, I, NI
Knife electrode					3, 5 mm, E		
Laser laparoscope sets			X				
Loop-tipped electrode				E	E	E, D	

*All instruments work through 5 mm ports unless otherwise indicated.

ABBREVIATIONS: A = atraumatic; B = bipolar; D = disposable; E = electrocautery; I = insulated; NI = not insulated; PDB = properitoneal dissection balloon; RT = ratchet; S = serrated; T = traumatic; U = unipolar; WS = with suction; WT = with teeth.

Marlow Surgical	Nortech	Olympus	Origin Medsystems	Storz	U.S. Surgical	Linvatec	Haraeus Surgical	Wolf
NI, I						NI		
NI, I				X	E, S, D	I		NI
				I, NI, 5, 10 mm	E, D	E, 10 mm		
NI, I				NI, 10 mm	D, T, NI, RT, 10 mm	NI, 10 mm		E
S, NI, I				I, NI		E	I, NI	E, 3, 5 mm
S, NI, I				I, NI		E	I, NI	E
		NI			D, A, NI, RT, 10 mm		NI	
NI, 5, 10, 11 mm	NI, 5, 10 mm	NI, 5, 11 mm		NI, 5, 10 mm		NI, 10 mm	NI	NI, 10 mm
		E		E	E, D			
		E	S, D, B, I, 33, 45 cm	E			E, WS	
E, WS		E, 4, 5 mm		B, U	X	E	E	E
NI, I				I, NI, U, 5, 10 mm	E, D	I, NI		
NI, E		NI	D, E, U, I	I, NI, U, 5, 10 mm	E, D			
E				A, B, E, I, NI, U, 5, 10 mm	D, I	I, NI	E	
					X			
					X			
NI, I		E					E	E
S, NI, E	NI	NI		I, E, RT	E, D	NI, I	NI	E
NI, I	E	NI		I, E	D, T, NI, RT	NI, I	NI	E
NI, I						3, 4 prong		
E	E, WS	E, 4, 5 mm		E	X	E	E	E
NI, E	E	4, 5 mm, I		I, NI, U	D, NI	NI, I	NI, E	E
E		E		E	E, D		E	E
X		X						

Table A-4

Grasping, holding, cutting, coagulation, and retraction—cont'd

				Manufacturers			
Instrument	Advanced Surgical	Cabot Medical	Circon ACMI	Cook Urological	Elmed	Ethicon Endo-Surgery	Jarit
Maryland dissector		NI	E, I				E, I, 5, 10 mm
Micro dissecting forceps		NI	E, I				E, I
Micro scissors		E	E, I			E, D	NI
Needle nose dissector		E, RT	E, I				E, I
Right-angled dissector		NI					NI, 10 mm
Pencil-tipped electrode		E		E	E	E, D	
Spatula electrode, U		E	E, I		E	E, D	E, WS
Spoon forceps		NI					NI
Sponge holder							RT, 10 mm
Stone forceps, 11 mm		NI					NI, 10 mm
Straight scissors		S, E	E, I			E, D	S, NI
Straight scissors, 11 mm		NI, S			E		S, NI, 10 mm
Retractors	5, 10 mm	10 mm	10 mm	1 mm		E, D	5, 10 mm
PDB retractor/dissector							

Table A-5

Ligation and suturing*

				Manufacturers			
Instrument	Advanced Surgical	Cabot Medical	Cook Urological	Elmed	Ethicon Endo-Surgery	Jarit	Marlow Surgical
Applicator for ligature loop		X	X			5, 10 mm	X
Knot pusher	5 mm	X				5, 10 mm	X
Clips		10 mm			A, NA		
Clip applicator		S, 11 mm			S, M, 10 mm	S, 10 mm	
Ligature loop					X		X
Extracorporeal ligature					X		X
Needle holders		3, 5 mm	3, 5 mm			3, 5, 10 mm	3, 5 mm
Staplers					12, 18 mm		

*All instruments work through 5 mm ports unless otherwise indicated.
ABBREVIATIONS: A = absorbable; M = multiple clips; NA = nonabsorbable; S = single clip.

Manufacturers

Marlow Surgical	Nortech	Olympus	Origin Medsystems	Storz	U.S. Surgical	Linvatec	Haraeus Surgical	Wolf
E, NI, I		E		I, U				
NI, B	I	NI		I, U, RT			NI	NI
NI NI, I	I	NI		NI	E, D	I	NI	NI
E								
		E		I, U, E				
E	E, WS	E		I, E	X	E	E	
NI, E, 10, 11 mm	NI, 10 mm	NI, 11 mm		NI, 10 mm			NI	NI, 5, 10 mm
NI, I, 10 mm							NI	
NI, I, 10 mm								
S, NI, I, E			D, E, U, I, RH	I, NI, U NI	E, D D, I, U	NI	S, NI	S, E NI, S
		10 mm		5, 10 mm	D, A, I, 10 mm			10 mm
			Gasless					

Manufacturers

Nortech	Olympus	Origin Medsystems	Storz	U.S. Surgical	Linvatec	Haraeus Surgical	Wolf
X	X		X	X		X	X
			X	X			
	NA		NA	X	NA	A, NA	
	S, 11 mm	M, NA, 10 mm	S, 11 mm	M, 10 mm	S, 10 mm	S, 11 mm	
			X	A, NA		X	
X	X		X	A, NA		X	X
3, 5 mm	3, 5 mm		3, 5 mm	NA 12, 15 mm GIA, TA, vascular, tissue	3, 5 mm	3, 5 mm	3, 5 mm

Table A-6 — Organ entrapment and morcellation*

	Manufacturers									
Instrument	Cabot Medical	Cook Urological	Dexide	Elmed	Ethicon Endo-Surgery	Olympus	Storz	U.S. Surgical	Haraeus Surgical	Wolf
Organ entrapment sack	10 mm 2 × 7 in	12 mm 2 × 5 in 5 × 8 in	10 mm 2 × 5 in 3 × 6 in 5 × 8 in		10 mm 4 × 4 in 2.5 × 6 in			10 mm		
Morcellator		PD, 11 mm		HD, 11 mm		HD, 11 mm	HD, 11 mm		HD, 11 mm	HD, 11 mm

*All instruments work through 5 mm ports unless otherwise indicated.
ABBREVIATIONS: HD = hand driven; PD = power driven.

Table A-7 — Aspiration and irrigation*

	Manufacturers						
Instrument	Cabot Medical	Circon ACMI	Cook Urological	Dexide	Elmed	Ethicon Endo-Surgery	Jarit
Aqua/hydro dissection probe	X	X					
Aspiration/injection needle	X	X	X		X	D, E	X
Aspiration/irrigation probe, single valve	X		10 mm		3, 5 mm, E		E, HE, SE, ND
Aspiration/irrigation probe, dual valve	D, ND	HE, SE			3, 5 mm		5, 10 mm
Aspiration/irrigation probe, triple valve		X			3, 5, 8 mm, PS		
Aspirator/irrigator system	X	1-5 L/min		D	3, 5, 11 mm, E		
Irrigation pump	X				CO_2 driven		
Suction/irrigation probe				D			

*All instruments work through 5 mm ports unless otherwise indicated.
ABBREVIATIONS: D = disposable; E = with coagulating electrode; H = with hook; HE = with hook electrode; ND = nondisposable; PS = pool suction; SE = with spatula electrode.

| | Manufacturers | | | | | | | |
Laserscope	Marlow Surgical	Nortech	Olympus	Origin Medsystems	Storz	Linvatec	Haraeus Surgical	Wolf
	X				X		X	X
X	X	X			X	X	X	X
	HE	E, HE, SE	E, HE, SE			E, HE, SE	X	E, HE, SE
H	X	X		D, 5, 10 mm	X	X	X	
		X	X		E, HE, SE	X	X	
X	X		X		X, PS	1-3 L/min, CO_2 driven		
					0-775 mm Hg pressure		0-750 mm Hg pressure	X

Table A-8

Laparoscopic instrument manufacturers

Company	Address	Telephone no.	FAX no.	Special instruments
Advanced Surgical, Inc.	305 College Rd. East Princeton, NJ 08540	(800)842-0320	(609)987-2342	
American Hydro-Surgical Instruments	430 Commerce Dr Ste 50 E Delray Beach, FL 33445	(800)527-5294	(407)278-5358	
Apple Medical	93 Nashaway Rd. Bolton, MA 01740	(508)779-2926	(508)779-6927	
Applied Medical Resources	Bldg. 104 26051 Merit Circle Laguna Hills, CA 92653	(714)367-8500	(714)582-6243	
Aspen Labs	14603 E. Fremont Ave. Englewood, CO 80112	(800)552-0138	(303)699-9854	Electrosurgical generator
Baxter V. Mueller	1435 Lake Cook Rd. Deerfield, IL 60015	(708)647-9383		
Birtcher	50 Technology Dr. Irvine, CA 92718	(800)888-1771	(714)753-9171	Argon beam coagulator
Cabot Medical	2021 Cabot Blvd. West Langhorne, PA 19047	(800)523-6078 (215)752-8300	(215)750-0161	
Circon ACMI	300 Stillwater Ave. Stamford, CT 06902	(800)325-7107 (203)328-8689	(203)328-8789	
Coherent Medical	3270 W. Bayshore Rd. Palo Alto, CA 94303	(800)635-1313	(415)857-0146	
Cook Urological	1100 W. Morgan St. P.O. Box 227 Spencer, IN 47460	(800)457-4448 (812)829-4891	(812)829-2022	Entrapment sack, tissue morcellator
DaVinci Medical	13700 First Ave. N. Plymouth, MN 55441	(612)473-4245	(612)473-3203	DaVinci handle instruments
Dexide	7509 Flagstone Dr. Fort Worth, TX 76118	(800)645-3378	(817)595-3300	
Electroscope	4890 Sterling Dr. Boulder, CO 80301	(303)444-2600	(303)444-2693	Endpoint monitor for monopolar electrodes
Elmed	60 West Fay Ave. Addison, IL 60101	(708)543-2792	(708)543-2102	
ENDOlap	3012 Mercy Dr. Orlando, FL 32808	(407)295-9955	(407)295-9966	
EndoMedix Corp.	2132 Michelson Dr Irvine, CA 92715	(800)553-6361 (714)253-1050	(714)253-1111	LaproScan: laparoscopic ultrasonic imaging
Ethicon Endo-Surgery	4545 Creek Rd. Cincinnati, OH 45242-2839	(800)873-3636 (513)786-7000	(513)786-7080	
Fujinon, Inc.	10 High Point Dr. Wayne, NJ 07470	(201)633-5600	(201)633-5216	Flexible video laparoscopes
Haraeus Surgical	575 Cottonwood Dr. Miopitas, CA 95035	(800)227-8372	(408)954-4040	
Jarit Instruments	9 Skyline Dr. Hawthorne, NY 10532	(800)431-1123 (914)592-9050	(914)592-8056	Rotating, articulating instruments
Kirwan Surgical	83 East Water St. P.O. Box 545 Rockland, MA 02370	(617)871-1876	(617)871-2816	

Table A-8	Laparoscopic instrument manufacturers—cont'd			
Company	Address	Telephone no.	FAX no.	Special instruments
Laserscope	3052 Orchard Dr. San Jose, CA 95134	(800)356-7600 (408)943-0636	(408)943-1051	KTP/YAG surgical laser system
Linvatec	11311 Concept Blvd. Largo, FL 34643	(800)237-0169	(813)399-5256	
Marlow Surgical Technologies, Inc.	1810 Joseph Lloyd Parkway Willoughby, OH 44094	(800)992-5581 (216)946-2453	(216)946-1997	
Medical Dynamics	99 Inverness Dr. East Englewood, CO 80112	(800)525-1294 (303)790-2990	(303)799-1378	Electronic Video Laparoscope™, video imaging equipment
Merocel Corporation	950 Flanders Rd. Mystic, CT 06355-0334	(800)637-6235	(203)572-7485	Antifog solution, presaturated antifog sponge
MP Video	63 South St. Hopkinton, MA 01748	(800)624-6274 (508)435-2131	(508)435-2227	Video endoscopy
Nortech	3930 Ventura Dr. Arlington Heights, IL 60004	(800)451-0918 (718)506-9872	(708)506-9891	
Olympus	4 Nevada Dr. Lake Success, NY 11042-1179	(800)548-5515 (516)488-3880	(516)326-9085	
Origin Medsystems, Inc.	135 Constitution Dr. Menlo Park, CA 94025	(415)617-5000	(415)617-5100	Gasless laparoscopy systems, procedure kits
Performance Surgical Instruments	40 Norfolk Ave. S. Easton, MA 02375	(800)622-1223 (508)230-0010	(508)238-3807	
Snowden-Pencer	5175 S. Royal Atlanta Dr. Tucker, GA 30081	(404)496-0952	(414)934-4922	
Storz	600 Corporate Pointe Culver City, CA 90230	(800)421-0837 (310)558-1500	(310)280-2504	Hopkins telescopes, Take-Apart instruments
Stryker Endoscopy	210 Baypointe Parkway San Jose, CA 95134	(800)624-4422 (408)435-0220	(408)435-1888	
Surgical Laser Technologies, Inc.	200 Cresson Blvd. Oaks, PA 19456	(800)366-4758	(215)650-3208	
U.S. Surgical Corp.	150 Glover Ave. Norwalk, CT 06856	(800)722-USSC (203)845-1000	(203)544-USSC	Endoclip, Endostapler, Endoshears
Wolf	353 Corporate Woods Pky. Vernon Hills, IL 60061	(800)323-WOLF	(708)913-1488	

Patient Education Booklet

David M. Albala

LAPAROSCOPY: A VALUABLE PROCEDURE

Your physician has recommended laparoscopy because it is a relatively uncomplicated procedure involving minimal discomfort and a short hospital stay. You have already undergone several diagnostic tests, and laparoscopy will be the next step in diagnosing or treating your condition.

Translated from the Greek, "laparoscopy" means examination of the inside of the abdomen. Laparoscopy is a technique that involves the insertion of a slender, light-producing "telescope" into the abdomen to provide the surgeon with a direct view of the interior of the abdomen. Laparoscopy was originally used only as a diagnostic procedure, but now many operations are performed using laparoscopy. In laparoscopic surgery two to six very small incisions (less than ½ inch) are made in the abdomen. Through these incisions, small metal tubes can be placed to allow the surgeon to view the interior of the abdomen and pass instruments for performing surgery. This booklet will explain the general technique of laparoscopy and will help answer your questions about the procedure. If you have any questions about your laparoscopic surgery, please ask your physician.

PREPARATION BEFORE SURGERY

Before your laparoscopic procedure, you might undergo a bowel preparation and a few routine tests to assess your general health. You will be asked not to eat or drink anything after midnight preceding the day of your laparoscopy. If in the past you have bled for a long time from a minor operation such as tooth extraction, please be sure to tell your physician. If you are taking aspirin or any other blood thinner, you should notify your surgeon so its use can be stopped or altered before your procedure.

After you are admitted to the hospital or clinic, you will be asked to sign a consent form. Your physician will discuss the procedure with you and explain how laparoscopy is to be used in your individual case.

THE LAPAROSCOPIC PROCEDURE (HOW LAPAROSCOPY WORKS)

Laparoscopic surgery is usually performed in the operating room. You will first be given a general anesthetic; this allows you to sleep through the surgery and wears off shortly after the operation is concluded. A breathing tube is routinely placed so the anesthesiologist can regulate your breathing while you are asleep. Usually, a bladder catheter and nasogastric tube are placed after you are anesthetized to drain these organs and decrease the risk of injury to them. After the anesthetic has taken effect, your physician will inflate your abdomen with a gas (such as carbon dioxide), much like a balloon, to create a clear space to view the inside of the abdominal cavity. This is done by inserting a needle into the lower abdomen and filling the abdomen with carbon dioxide gas to lift the abdominal wall away from the organs. The next step in the procedure is to make a small incision (less than ½ inch) in the lower abdomen and insert a small hollow metal tube called a "trocar." Through this trocar, a laparoscope (a small telescope with lenses and a light) is passed, which allows the surgeon to see the interior of the abdomen. After the laparoscope is positioned, other small incisions may be made and additional trocars may be inserted. Special surgical instruments will be placed through these trocars that allow the surgeon to operate.

At the end of the procedure, the carbon dioxide gas is expelled from the abdomen and each small incision is stitched closed. You will then be moved into the recovery area until you awaken from the anesthetic.

RECOVERY FROM LAPAROSCOPY

After the procedure you will stay in the recovery area where specially trained nurses will monitor your progress. After a few hours you will either be allowed to go home or you will be moved to a regular hospital room. You will stay in the hospital for observation and recovery according to your needs as determined by your physician. During your recovery you may have some abdominal pain that can be relieved by oral pain medication. You may also feel some shoulder pain; this is caused by the carbon dioxide gas that was present in the upper abdomen. This pain usually disappears in a few hours after surgery. Once you are released from the hospital, you can resume your normal activities within a week or less, depending on your progress. The nurses will teach you how to care for your small incisions before you are discharged.

Do not be surprised if you notice some bruising around the incision sites 1 or 2 days after your discharge. Indeed, at times some blood may spread under the skin and cause the entire lower half of the abdomen to turn blue; however, this occurrence is usually of no significance. Nevertheless, you should notify your physician if this occurs. Usually over 3 to 5 days, the blue color turns yellow and then disappears.

During your recovery at home, be sure to call your physician immediately if you experience any severe abdominal pain, fever, or redness, swelling, and/or drainage from the incisions.

THE RISKS AND BENEFITS OF LAPAROSCOPY

Complications of laparoscopy, such as bleeding, infection, and injury to abdominal organs, occur infrequently. Your physician will discuss the risks of any possible complications based on your individual case. In some cases a standard open operation may become necessary. Your physician will make this decision in the operating room; this occurs in less than 5% of cases. However, you must realize that laparoscopy is *no guarantee* that you will not have *open* surgery; if a problem arises during the procedure, open surgery may be necessary to save your life!

Since laparoscopy is performed with only one to six very small incisions, you will not have the large incision typical of the standard open surgical procedure. Because of this, you may experience less pain and have a shorter hospital stay than after traditional open surgery. The length of time required for you to resume your normal activities will depend largely on the nature of your problem. You may feel like limiting some of your activities for at least 1 or 2 days after your procedure. It is best to avoid strenuous work or sports for 1 week. After the procedure your physician will discuss the results of your laparoscopy and answer any questions.

DISCHARGE INSTRUCTIONS FOR LAPAROSCOPIC SURGERY

1. *Do not drive.* If your procedure is being done on an outpatient basis, the drugs administered during your operation may make you feel dizzy, alter your sense of balance and fine muscle control, and slow your reaction time. A family member or friend should drive you home.

2. While recuperating, you may have unpredictable reactions to the anesthesia, ranging from practically *no symptoms* to possibly 3 to 4 days of *feeling tired*.
3. You may have a *sore throat* for the first 24 hours. This is a result of the breathing tube placed in your throat during the surgery.
4. *Shoulder pain or chest pain* may occur during the first 3 to 4 hours following your procedure. However, if the discomfort lasts longer than a few hours or if you develop shoulder or chest pain after you have gone home, call your physician! This pain is caused by gas remaining in the abdomen. The gas irritates your abdominal wall, and this irritation may also be felt in your shoulders. If you are particularly uncomfortable, your pain may be relieved by lying flat and applying a heating pad to your shoulder.
5. Your arm may be sore at the intravenous needle site. Warm soaks (i.e., towels soaked in warm water and applied to the site) will help relieve this pain.
6. You may notice some *bruising across your abdomen*. This is a result of the insertion of the trocars during the surgical procedure and will disappear like any other bruise. The result may be that your entire abdomen turns blue. This blue color will fade over several days and then turn a dull yellow before disappearing completely.
7. The *bandages* on the skin openings should be left in place for 1 to 2 days. After this time they can be removed. The incisions can then be treated as any other cut on the skin. It is safe to shower or bathe the morning after your procedure.
8. *Full physical activity* should be delayed for 2 to 3 days.

Call the hospital emergency department or your physician should any of the following arise after you have left the hospital:
1. Fever higher than 100° F
2. Abdominal swelling
3. Intense or progressively worsening abdominal pain
4. Bleeding from one of the incisions
5. Chest or shoulder pain

Informed Consent

Howard N. Winfield

Overview

Every human being of adult years and sound mind has a right to determine what shall be done with his own body, and a surgeon who performs an operation without his patient's consent commits an assault for which he is liable in damages.

Justice Benjamin Cardozo, 1914

Laparoscopic surgery has created a multitude of new operative procedures that may now be offered to the patient. The advantages over traditional open surgery are decreased postoperative discomfort, hospitalization, and time of convalescence. This "minimally invasive" form of surgery creates small, cosmetically acceptable surgical scars. The financial savings appear to benefit the patient and, depending on the complexity of the procedure, may also benefit the third-party insurance carriers.

The disadvantages of laparoscopic surgery, as it is currently performed, are: (1) the operative site is approached by a transperitoneal route; thus there is the risk of injuring gastrointestinal, vascular, or other visceral structures within the peritoneal cavity, (2) the duration of the procedures is usually longer than for open surgery, (3) the learning curve is steep, and (4) the hospital's cost to purchase laparoscopic equipment and the surgeon's cost to attend training seminars are significant.

Therefore the patient who is scheduled for a laparoscopic procedure should be informed that laparoscopic surgery is relatively new and the surgeon performing the operation may have limited experience with the technique. In fact, the patient should be informed when he or she may be the surgeon's "first patient." An honest and open disclosure of the surgeon's experience with a given laparoscopic procedure is mandatory. The patient should be informed that at some point during the laparoscopy it may become apparent to the surgeon that the planned laparoscopic surgery may not be possible because of technical reasons, resulting in the need for traditional open surgery. The risks of vascular, intestinal, or other abdominal visceral injury may require emergency laparotomy. The potential of requiring a vascular graft, colostomy, splenectomy, or other ancillary procedure is remote but should be mentioned. Intraoperative anesthetic or pulmonary complications should be discussed. Finally, the patient should be told that the occurrence of uncontrollable hemorrhage may result in death.

Specific to each laparoscopic procedure, a clear description of the diagnosis and planned operation should be discussed with the patient. Alternative methods of therapy should also be described.

With careful counseling of the patient before embarking on laparoscopic procedures, the potential for confrontation with medicolegal issues can be significantly diminished. However, the surgeon should always bear in mind that *"the law does not allow a crime to be licensed by a victim's consent."*

GENERAL INFORMED CONSENT FOR ALL LAPAROSCOPIC PROCEDURES
I have elected to undergo my surgery by means of a laparoscopic approach. I understand there are certain risks common to all laparoscopic procedures.

1. I understand that I will be given a general anesthestic. The potential risks of general anesthesia are generally minor in nature, including nausea or vomiting, lethargy or headache, and a sore throat from the breathing tube that is used during the procedure. However, I understand that other more serious problems can occur with the heart and lungs, such as heart attacks, low blood pressure, pneumonia, and blood clots in the legs or lungs; although rare, these potential complications can even result in death.

2. To perform laparoscopy, I understand that it is usually necessary to fill my abdomen with a gas such as carbon dioxide or nitrous oxide. As a result, the gas may collect beneath the tissues of the skin. If this occurs, the collection of gas usually will disappear within 24 hours of my surgery.

I also understand that sometimes the retained carbon dioxide may result in temporary shoulder pain after surgery, usually resolving within 24 hours.

Although rare, more serious problems that can arise from introducing gas into my abdomen include blood abnormalities that might result in raising or lowering of my blood pressure, abnormal heartbeats, or the anesthesiologist's inability to breathe for me while I am asleep.

Last, I understand that there is a rare risk of death from the use of gas to expand my abdomen. This can occur if a large amount of gas enters one of my blood vessels and advances to the lung or causes an abnormal heartbeat.

3. To perform laparoscopy, I understand that it is necessary for the surgeon to pass sharpened hollow metal or plastic tubes into my abdomen. Passage of these tubes may result in bruising of the skin. I understand that this bruising sometimes can be quite extensive but will usually resolve within 2 to 3 weeks after the procedure.

I also understand that during the placement of any of these tubes, injury can occur to a blood vessel or to an organ within my abdomen. If this happens, I understand that I may need open surgery to repair the damage. I also understand that this type of problem could lead to severe infection, low blood pressure, the need for blood transfusion, and even death.

I also understand that the liver, colon, spleen, stomach, small bowel or intestine, gallbladder, or urinary bladder may be injured during the procedure, which may require open surgical repair.

4. If postoperative bleeding, bowel perforation, ureteral or bladder injury, or infection would be recognized, I understand that additional therapy, a longer hospitalization, and possibly even a subsequent open operation may be necessary. I understand that these complications can result in my death.

5. I understand that even though the incisions in my abdomen are small, they can be painful and become infected. I also understand that there is risk that a piece of my bowel may bulge through these incisions after surgery. If this occurs, I may require a separate operation to repair the incisional defect (hernia).

6. I understand that, although extremely rare, injury from positioning during surgery can occur that may cause temporary or permanent weakness or numbness in my arms, hands, or legs.

7. I understand that if the laparoscopic procedure cannot be done because of technical or anatomic problems, open incisional surgery may be necessary.

Periprocedural Order Sheet

David M. Albala

PREPROCEDURE ORDERS FOR LAPAROSCOPY

☐ Condition: _____

_____

☐ Diagnosis: _____

_____

☐ Allergies: _____

_____

☐ Activity: Ad lib
☐ Diet: NPO after midnight
☐ IV: Start D_5 ½ NS with 20 mEq KCL at 80 cc/hr at 8 AM
☐ Premedications: _____

_____

☐ Medications
   GoLYTELY or NuLYTELY, 4 to 6 L PO, starting at 1 PM
   Neomycin, 2 g at 7 PM and 11 PM before the day of surgery
   Compazine, 10 mg PO at 2 PM to stop nausea
   Metronidazole, 2 g at 7 PM and 11 PM before the day of surgery
   Ancef, 1 g IV on call to OR
☐ Labs: Routine admission plus PT/PTT, platelets; type and screen (for diagnostic or minor therapeutic laparoscopy); cross-match for 2 units (for major therapeutic laparoscopy)
☐ Notify on-call resident if: _____

_____

_____

POSTPROCEDURE ORDERS FOR LAPAROSCOPY

☐ Condition: _____

_____

☐ Diagnosis: _____

_____

☐ Allergies: _____

_____

☐ Activity: Ad lib
☐ Diet: Clear liquids; advance as tolerated
☐ IV: D_5 ½ NS with 20 mEq KCL at 100 cc/hr; D/C when oral intake is well tolerated
☐ Medications
    Ancef, 1 g IV q 8 × 24 hr, then begin
    Keflex, 250 mg PO q 6 × 24 hr
    Tylenol #3, 1 to 2 tablets PO q 4-6 hr prn for pain
☐ Laboratory workup: CBC in AM
☐ Intake and output
☐ Notify on-call resident if: _____

_____

_____

SAGES Guidelines for Granting of Privileges for Laparoscopic (Peritoneoscopic) General Surgery

PRINCIPLES OF PRIVILEGING

Preamble

The Society of American Gastrointestinal Endoscopic Surgeons recommends the following guidelines for privileging qualified surgeons in the performance of general surgical procedures utilizing laparoscopy (cholecystectomy, appendectomy, hernia repair and other similar procedures). The basic premise is that the surgeon must have the judgment, training and the capability of immediately proceeding to a traditional open abdominal procedure when circumstances so indicate.

This document is to serve as a guide for granting privileges in laparoscopic surgery as an integral part of surgical practice. Surgeons who are experienced in operating upon abdominal organs are familiar with anatomy, tissue tolerance, organ compliance and pathological processes and should readily develop laparoscopic proficiency which should be assessed regardless of the number of procedures performed.

Purpose

The purpose of this statement is to outline principles and provide practical suggestions to assist hospital privileging committees when granting privileges to perform laparoscopic surgery. In conjunction with the standard JCAHO guidelines for granting hospital privileges, implementation of these methods should help hospital staffs ensure that laparoscopic surgery is performed only by individuals with appropriate

Reprinted by permission of the Society of Gastrointestinal Endoscopic Surgeons (SAGES). SAGES guidelines. Surg Endosc 7:67-68, 1993.

competence, thus assuring high quality patient care and proper procedure utilization.

Uniformity of standards

Uniform standards should be developed which apply to all hospital staff requesting privileges to perform laparoscopic general surgery. Criteria must be established which are medically sound but not unreasonably stringent and which are universally applicable to all those wishing to obtain privileges. The goal must be the delivery of high quality patient care.

Responsibility for privileging

The privileging structure and process remain the individual responsibility of each hospital. It should be the responsibility of the Department of Surgery, through its Chief, to recommend individual surgeons for privileges in laparoscopic general surgery as for other procedures performed by members of the department.

TRAINING AND DETERMINATION OF COMPETENCE
Formal fellowship or residency training in general surgery
Determination of competence in laparoscopic surgery

A surgical residency/fellowship program which incorporates structured experience in laparoscopic surgery should be completed. The applicant's Program Director or laparoscopic training director should confirm in writing the training, experience and actual observed level of competency as is done for other procedures in general surgery.

The surgeon should demonstrate proficiency in laparoscopic surgical procedures and clinical judgment equivalent to that obtained in a residency/fellowship program. Documentation and demonstration of competence is necessary with verification in writing from experienced colleagues.

For those without residency training or fellowship which included laparoscopic surgery or without documented prior experience in laparoscopic surgery, the process should be similar to a residency experience including didactics, hands-on animal experience, participation as a first assistant and performance of the operation under proctorship. The basic minimum requirements for training should be:

1. Completion of approved residency training in general surgery, with privileging in the comparable open procedure for which laparoscopic privileges are being sought.
2. Privileging in diagnostic laparoscopy.

3. Training in laparoscopic general surgery by a surgeon experienced in laparoscopic surgery or completion of a university sponsored or academic society recognized didactic course which includes instruction in handling and use of laparoscopic instrumentation, principles of safe trocar insertion, establishment of safe peritoneal access, laparoscopic tissue handling, knot tying, equipment utilization (e.g., staplers), as well as animal experience in specific categories of procedures for which applicant desires privileges. The individual must demonstrate to the satisfaction of an experienced physician course director/preceptor that he/she can perform a given procedure from beginning to end in an animal model. Such proficiency for each category of procedure in question must be documented in writing by the physician course director. The course content and procedures taught should clearly include material specific to the category of procedure for which privileges are sought. Attendance at short courses which do not provide supervised hands-on training or documentation of proficiency is not an acceptable substitute.

4. Experience as first assistant to a previously privileged individual performing the category of the laparoscopic procedures for which privileges are being sought in patients; documentation to be provided by the privileged individual.

5. Proctoring by a laparoscopic surgeon experienced in the same or similar procedure(s) until proficiency has been observed and documented in writing.

Proctoring

Recognizing the limitations of written reports, proctoring of applicants for privileges in laparoscopic surgery by a qualified, unbiased staff surgeon experienced in general and laparoscopic surgery is recommended. The procedural details of proctoring should be developed by the privileging body of the hospital and provided to the applicant. Proctors may be chosen from existing staff or solicited from surgical endoscopic societies. The proctor should be responsible to the privileging committee, and not to the patient or to the individual being proctored. Documentations of the proctor's evaluation should be submitted in writing to the privileging committee. Criteria of competency for each procedure should be established in advance and should include evaluation of: familiarity with instrumentation and equipment, competence in their use, appropriateness of patient selection, clarity of dissection, safety, time taken to complete the procedure and successful completion of same. It is essential that proctoring be provided in an unbiased, confidential and objective manner. A satisfactory mechanism for appeal must be established for individuals whom privileges are denied or granted in a temporary or provisional manner.

Monitoring of laparoscopic performance

To assist the hospital privileging body in the ongoing renewal of privileges, there should be a mechanism for monitoring each surgical laparoscopist's procedural performance. This should be done through existing quality assurance mechanisms. This should include monitoring utilization, diagnostic and therapeutic benefits to patients, complications and tissue review in accordance with previously developed criteria.

Continuing education

Continuing medical education related to laparoscopic surgery should be required as part of the periodic renewal of privileges. Attendance at appropriate local or national meetings and courses is encouraged.

Renewal of privileges

For the renewal of privileges an appropriate level of continuing clinical activity should be required. In addition to satisfactory performance as assessed by monitoring of procedural activity through existing quality assurance mechanisms, continuing medical education relating to laparoscopic surgery should also be required.

Acknowledgments   This statement was reviewed and approved by the Board of Governors of the Society of American Gastrointestinal Endoscopic Surgeons (SAGES) October, 1992. It was prepared by the SAGES Committee on Credentialing.

REFERENCES

1. SAGES. Granting of privileges for laparoscopic general surgery. Am J Surg 161:324-325, 1991.
2. Dent TL. Clinical privileges for laparoscopic general surgery. Am J Surg 161:399-403, 1991.
3. Greene FL. Training, credentialing and privileging for minimally invasive surgery. Prob Gen Surg 8:502-506, 1991.
4. New York State Department of Health Memorandum. Laparoscopic Surgery. Series 92-20, Albany, New York, June 12, 1992.

Index